# What Doctors Don't Know about Breastfeeding

Jack Newman, MD, IBCLC, FRCPC
Andrea Polokova, MA, IBCLC

Praeclarus Press, LLC
©2022 Jack Newman and Andrea Polokova.

www.PraeclarusPress.com

Praeclarus Press, LLC
2504 Sweetgum Lane
Amarillo, Texas 79124 USA
806-367-9950
www.PraeclarusPress.com

**DISCLAIMER**

The information contained in this publication is advisory only and is not intended to replace sound clinical judgment or individualized patient care. The author disclaims all warranties, whether expressed or implied, including any warranty as the quality, accuracy, safety, or suitability of this information for any particular purpose.

ISBN: 978-1-946665-56-0

Cover Design: Ken Tackett
Developmental Editing: Kathleen Kendall-Tackett
Copyediting: Chris Tackett

Layout & Design: Nelly Murariu

# CONTENTS

*Introduction*                                                              ix

## SECTION I: The Fundamentals                                              1

### 1:  A Short History of Infant Feeding                                   3
Hunter/Gatherer Societies                                                   3
Wet Nursing                                                                 4
The Advent of Commercial Infant Formula                                     6
Formula Companies Keep Up Disinformation                                    9
Conclusion                                                                 11

### 2:  Medical Education and Breastfeeding                                13
What Passes for Medical Education about Breastfeeding                      13
Common Myths that Health Professionals Believe                            17
Not Enough Milk                                                           18
How Things Have *Not* Changed!                                            19

### 3:  Is Formula the Same as Breastmilk?                                 21
"New and Improved"                                                        22
What Formula Lacks                                                        25
Breastmilk Also Varies by Time of Day                                     27
Breastmilk Varies by the Child's Age                                      27
Commercial Infant Formula and the Microbiome                             28
Do Studies Show Any Real Difference?                                      29
Conclusion                                                               30

### 4:  The Right to Breastfeed                                            31
System Failures Force Mothers to Use Formula                              31
Breastfeeding and Legal Issues                                           33
Conclusion                                                               35

## Section II: The Postpartum Period 37

**5: Is Breastfeeding Risky?** 39
The Media and Breastfeeding 40
Conclusions 43

**6: Birth Interventions** 45
Intravenous Fluids 45
Epidurals 46
The Breast Crawl and Skin to Skin 48
Kangaroo Mother Care (KMC) 49
Conclusions 50

**7: Dehydration and Weight Loss after Birth** 51
10% Loss of Birthweight: The Gold Standard? 54
Observing Babies at the Breast: The Better Metric 58
When Supplementation Is Necessary 59
Conclusion 61

**8: Hypoglycemia** 63
Maternal Diabetes as a Risk Factor 63
Large (or Small) for Gestational Age 64
Blood Glucose Normally Drops 65
Nature Provides a Backup Plan: Ketone Bodies 66
No Need to Separate Mothers at Risk for Low Blood Glucose 66
Prenatal Expression of Colostrum 67
Conclusion 68

**9: High Bilirubin and Jaundice** 69
Hemolysis 69
Monitoring Bilirubin 70
"Breastmilk Jaundice" 72
Biliary Atresia: Important to Rule Out 74
Gilbert's Syndrome 75
What Is the Bottom Line? 75

# Section III: Latching On and Drinking Well      77

**10:  Latch and Drinking at the Breast**                      79
Sore Nipples Are *Not* a Normal Part of Breastfeeding          80
What to Do for Sore Nipples                                    82
How to Evaluate Latch                                          84
How to Know If the Baby Is Drinking at the Breast              85
What to Do When Babies Are Not Drinking Well                   90
Conclusion                                                     93

**11:  Breast Pain, Infection, and Lumps**                     95
Engorgement                                                    95
Blocked Ducts and Mastitis                                     97
Breast Abscess                                                 99
Who Should Treat a Breast Abscess?                             101
Galactocele                                                    105
Investigating a Lump in the Breast                             108
Conclusion                                                     111

**12:  Tongue-Tie**                                            113
Tongue-Tie Alone May Not Be a Problem                          114
An Anecdote                                                    115
Diagnosing Tongue-Tie                                          116
Releasing Tongue-Ties                                          121
Tongue-Tie Release and Domperidone                             124
What About Upper Lip Ties?                                      124
Conclusion                                                     125

**13:  Nipple Shields**                                        127
The Problem with Nipple Shields                                127
What Could Be Done Instead?                                    132
Conclusions                                                    133

## Section IV: Milk Supply     135

### 14: Is the Baby Getting Enough to Eat? Assessing Infant Weight Gain   137
What Happens When Doctors Are Concerned?   137
What Healthcare Providers Should Do Instead   139
Growth Curves   140
Exclusively Breastfed Babies Can Grow and Thrive   145
Managing Slow Weight Gain   147
Can a Baby Gain Too Much?   149
Is Serum Sodium a Good Measure Baby's Intake?   152
Conclusion   153

### 15: Late Onset Decreasing Milk Supply and Flow   155
It's Not an Allergy   158
Causes of Late Onset Decreasing Milk Supply and Flow   160
Symptoms of Late Onset Decreasing Milk Supply and Flow   163
Prevention   170
Treatment   170
Conclusion   172

### 16: Domperidone   173
Using Domperidone   173
Possible Side Effects of Domperidone   176
Most Doctors Do Not Know about Domperidone   177
Options for Domperidone   178
Domperidone Paranoia   178
Our Response to the Health Canada Warnings   180
Conclusion   182

### 17: Relactation   183
Why Are Mothers Unnecessarily Told to Stop Breastfeeding?   183
What Can Be Done?   184
Conclusion   188

### 18: Inducing Lactation   189
Reasons for Inducing Lactation   189
How to Induce Lactation   190

Medications We Recommend for Inducing Lactation 191
Six to 8 Weeks Before the Baby Is Due 192
When To Put the Baby to the Breast 193
Should the Birth Mother Breastfeed? 194
When the Parents Are Two Women and One Is Pregnant 195
Follow-Up 195
Case Study 196

# Section V: Mothers' Health — 199

## 19: When Mothers Are Sick — 201
Infectious Diseases 201
Common Infectious Diseases and Breastfeeding 203
Hepatitis 206
Non-Infectious Diseases 213
Conclusions 213

## 20: Maternal Medications and Breastfeeding — 215
How Drugs Pass into Milk 215
Non-Useful Sources 217
There Are Risks Associated with Not Breastfeeding 218
Does Interrupting Breastfeeding Qualify as *Non Nocere* (Do No Harm)? 219
Medications that Never Enter Milk 219
Some Antibiotics Enter Milk but Babies Do Not Absorb Them 222
Radioactive Iodine is Contraindicated 223
Hormonal Contraception 225
Fertility Treatments 226
Ectopic Pregnancy 227
Conclusion 227

# Section VI: Infancy and Beyond — 229

## 21: Starting the Baby on Food — 231
What about Choking? 233
What about Breastfeeding? 235

Food Products That Breastfed Babies Do Not Need 235
When Older Babies Stop Gaining Weight—Ketosis 240
Conclusion 241

## 22: Infant Sleep and Sleep Training 243
What is Normal Infant Sleep? 244
Breastsleeping 245
Babies Need Contact with Their Mothers 246
Why Sleep-Deprived Parents Turn to Formula 247
How Breastfeeding Mothers Can Cope with Fatigue 248
This, Too, Shall Pass 250
When Doctors Recommend Sleep Training 252
Conclusion 253

## 23: How Long Is It Normal to Breastfeed? 255
Is Breastfeeding Past One Year Harmful? 255
Conclusion 263

## 24: Breastfeeding Myths That Even Some Lactation Consultants Believe 265
1. Babies Transfer Milk (No, They Do Not) 265
2. "Oversupply" is Common 268
3. Pumping Accurately Measures Supply 269
4. Test Weighing Is a Good Way to Know If the Baby Is Getting Enough 269
5. Breastmilk in a Bottle Is the Same as Breastfeeding 271
Conclusion 272

References 273

# Introduction

Physicians often lack even the most basic understanding of breastfeeding. This is true not only for general practitioners and pediatricians, but for health professionals in *all* medical specialties, including, bizarrely, specialists in pediatric nutrition. Indeed, one can confidently say that most physicians know so little about breastfeeding that they do not know what they do not know.

This lack of understanding influences how they discuss breastfeeding with mothers, their families, their colleagues, and the media. When breastfeeding problems arise, they do not know how to help the families and are often quick to tell mothers to stop and bottle-feed formula. Of course, this is not true of *all* physicians, but those who do know something about practical breastfeeding are a minority and those who know enough to counsel mothers are a minority within a minority.

Why do physicians know so little about something that seems essential to good care?

## Lack of Training

Lack of training is one problem. Breastfeeding is just simply not a formal part of health professionals' training: not during their undergraduate training, nor in their post-graduate training. Indeed, who is going to teach them? The previous generation of health professionals? They were also never taught about normal infant feeding and how to advise mothers on breastfeeding (Lien & Shattuck, 2017).

Even doctors who know about breastfeeding may not have practical knowledge, such as how to help mothers to latch their babies on as well as possible, the single most important skill a helper can have. Forget it! Formula and bottle-feeding are the usual answers, even when breastfeeding problems are easily solvable. The quick resort to formula and bottles also reflects a mindset that formula is a good substitute, and in some cases, are even better than breastfeeding itself. Children fed only formula usually grow up to be healthy, intelligent, and good people, right? Of course! Yet lack of breastfeeding increases health risks for both mothers and babies, and that part of the equation is rarely considered.

## Bottle-Feeding Influences

The more insidious issue, in our view, is that formula-feeding norms influence the very models of normal feeding. Take, for example, how often should a baby be fed? The bottle-fed, formula-fed baby receives a given amount of milk every 3 to 4 hours. The quantity of milk the baby drank is guaranteed (unless the baby is a habitual spitter upper). You can see exactly how much the baby drank. If the baby took 90 ml (3 oz) of milk every 3 hours, say, in accordance with the universally determined calculations (The baby needs to drink 150 cc/kg/day or 2.5 oz/lb/day), the baby should gain 30 grams/day (1 oz/day) for the first 3 or 4 months, and then 15 g/day (0.5 ounce/day) thereafter until 6 months. After 6 months, even less weight gain per day is considered acceptable. By 4 months of age, in accordance with pediatric teaching until a couple of decades ago, babies were started on "solid food" and the concern about how much milk they were drinking became even less of an issue. If the baby gained weight according to these guidelines, then the baby was probably healthy and taking in enough food (including formula). The "formula," based on the numbers, worked for most babies, but did not apply to the breastfed baby.

## Why This Matters

Unfortunately, physicians' lack of knowledge means that many mothers stop breastfeeding early, often much earlier than they had planned. There are enormous implications for this. Mothers often grieve when breastfeeding fails and they are more likely to become depressed (Borra, Iacovou, & Sevilla, 2015; A. E. Brown, 2019). And there are the risks of not breastfeeding.

## The Risks of Not Breastfeeding

Even though it is not politically correct to say, we need to acknowledge that mothers and babies are more prone to illness if breastfeeding does not work, or if babies are not breastfed as long as desirable and recommended (exclusive breastfeeding to 6 months with food added and continued breastfeeding to 2 years and beyond). Even those denying the "benefits" of breastfeeding have probably observed that breastfed babies are less likely to get diarrhea due to infections, especially if they are *exclusively* breastfed. Or that breastfed (or breastmilk fed) premature babies are less likely to get necrotizing enterocolitis, a very serious disorder of the intestinal tract that causes parts of the small and large intestine to die, with resulting lifelong problems of the intestinal tract (including insufficient absorption of nutrients).

Those discounting the value of breastfeeding do not think it is a big deal for babies in rich or industrialized nations like the United States, Canada, and Western Europe. They may dismiss necrotizing enterocolitis as a problem *only* for premature babies and argue that babies in "clean" countries like Canada, or other industrialized nations, are less likely to get intestinal infections. We note that necrotizing enterocolitis is indeed a big deal in that it is the most common cause of morbidity and death in premature babies, as well as lifelong ill health. Further, infectious diarrhea can be serious and commonly results in hospitalization and even death, even in first-world countries. Below is a partial research summary on the risks of not breastfeeding. Breastfeeding protects infants from:

- Diarrheal and respiratory infections (Duijts, Jaddoe, Hofman, & Moll, 2010; Li, Dee, Li, Hoffman, & Grummer-Strawn, 2014; Quigley, Kelly, & Sacker, 2007)
- Enterovirus infections (Sadeharju et al., 2007)
- Lower respiratory tract infections (Tromp et al., 2017)
- Overweight and obesity (Armstrong, Reilly, & The Child Health Information Team, 2002; Liese et al., 2001; W. Oddy, 2012, 2017; Yan, Liu, Zhu, Huang, & Wang, 2014)

- Psychosocial stress from parents' divorce (Montgomery, Ehlin, & Sacker, 2006)

- Mental health problems in adolescence (W. H. Oddy et al., 2009)

- Sudden infant death syndrome and infant mortality (Bartick & Reinhold, 2010; Thompson et al., 2017; Vennemann et al., 2009)

- Cognitive and learning problems (Quigley et al., 2012)

Breastfeeding also protects mothers from various diseases including:

- Breast cancer (Collaborative Group on Hormonal Factors in Breast Cancer, 2002; Tryggvadottir, Tulinius, Eyfjord, & Sigurvinsson, 2001), even with BRCA1 and BRCA2 mutations (Jernstrom et al., 2004)

- Ovarian cancer (Babic et al., 2020; Su, Pasalich, Lee, & Binns, 2013; Titus-Ernstoff et al., 2001; Tung et al., 2003)

- Type 2 diabetes (Gunderson et al., 2015; Ram et al., 2008; Stuebe, Rich-Edwards, Willett, Manson, & Michels, 2005)

- Cardiovascular disease (Schwartz et al., 2009)

## Health Organization Recommendations

Because of breastfeeding's key role in disease prevention, public-health organizations, such as the World Health Organization, the American Academy of Pediatrics, and UNICEF (the United Nations Children's Fund), unequivocally support breastfeeding. Below are recommendations from a document called the *Innocenti Declaration*, co-authored by WHO and UNICEF. (See Appendix A to read the full declaration.)

> WHO and UNICEF recommend that children initiate breastfeeding *within the first hour of birth* (our emphasis) and be exclusively breastfed for the first 6 months of life – meaning no other foods or liquids are provided, including water …
>
> Infants should be breastfed on demand – that is as often as the child wants, day and night. No bottles, teats or pacifiers should be used …

From the age of 6 months, children should begin eating safe and adequate complementary foods while continuing to breastfeed for up to 2 years and beyond.

These recommendations were reiterated in a recent joint statement on protecting maternal and child nutrition in the Ukraine war and refugee crisis (UNICEF, Global Nutrition Cluster, & IFE Core Group, 2022).

UNICEF, the Global Nutrition Cluster, and Partners call for ALL involved in the response to the Ukraine Conflict Crisis to protect, promote, and support the feeding and care of infants and young children and their caregivers. This is critical to support child survival, growth, and development and to prevent malnutrition, illness, and death.

## Why Aren't More Mothers Breastfeeding According to WHO Guidelines?

Major health organizations recommend that mothers breastfeed exclusively for at least 6 months, and then combine solid foods with continued breastfeeding up to age 2 *and beyond*. Unfortunately, most mothers, particularly in industrialized countries, do not reach these goals. Given these clear recommendations, why aren't more mothers breastfeeding according to these WHO guidelines. There are many reasons, but principally, we've identified four key factors:

### The Medical System Undermines Mothers' Ability to Breastfeed

We cover this in detail throughout the book, but medical practitioners' influence begins during pregnancy. Many doctors do not promote breastfeeding because they don't want mothers to feel guilty or because they do not consider breastfeeding important.

### The Belief That Artificial Infant Feeding Is Just as Good

Culture also has a role. Whole groups of people in many industrialized countries believe that formula is just as good as breastfeeding. A health professional who believes this often does so on the basis of personal or their spouse's experience. Family, friends, workplaces, and daycare providers subtly, or directly pressure the mother not to breastfeed, or to breastfeed only for a short time.

## The Insidious Influence of Formula Companies in Medical Education and "Free Gifts"

Formula generates billions in sales every year and formula manufacturers know just how to get their products to their key market. They bombard doctors and mothers with advertisements and "free gifts." Formula companies even give away attractive breastfeeding informational materials. Unfortunately, the underlying message of their materials is that breastfeeding usually doesn't work out (and here's a coupon for our product "just in case").

Formula companies also influence the education that doctors, especially pediatricians, receive. Advertising for pediatricians constantly tells them about the advantages of various formulas, including the highly profitable *special* formulas. If there is a problem, formula will solve it. Formula reps market their product in doctors' offices, at conferences, and even, shockingly, in conference sessions where nutrition or pediatric experts shill for the formula companies under the guise of professional education. The financial cooperation between medical education and formula companies has been condemned since the 1930s, yet continues today (Bognar et al., 2020).

## Lack of Maternity Leave

Mothers in many countries have little paid maternity leave. Three or four months is typical. In some cases, it doesn't exist at all. The U.S., for example, has no guaranteed maternity leave. Some individual companies offer it, and it is now available for federal workers, but one article reported that 25% of workers in the U.S. were returning to work at 2 weeks postpartum (Lerner, 2015).

Healthcare professionals should be at the forefront in the push for decent, paid maternity leave. In our opinion, anything less than 6 months *paid* maternity leave is completely inadequate; 1 year is much more reasonable because by one year, almost all babies can drink from an open cup and can have mother's expressed milk mixed with the baby's food. Thus, there is no need for bottles. We believe, for example, that the U.S. government made a huge mistake when it arranged for mothers to get free pumps to "support breastfeeding" instead of legislating reasonable maternity leave for all mothers.

## After Almost 50 Years, What Do We Still Not Know?

Unfortunately, even after 50 years of increasing breastfeeding rates, healthcare providers still do not understand some important principles about basic breastfeeding management. We will describe these throughout this book, but here are a few principles to get us started.

### Breastfeeding Should Not Hurt

Nipple pain is the most common reason why mothers stop breastfeeding early. Can you blame them? Pain is a sign that something is wrong, but many health professionals believe that it is a normal part of breastfeeding and, as a result, often do nothing besides telling mothers to "keep at it."

## The First Few Days After Birth Are *Crucial* to Get Breastfeeding Going Well

In many hospitals, babies are still routinely supplemented with formula. Some mothers and babies manage to breastfeed, but routine supplementation sabotages many. When mothers are disappointed by their breastfeeding experiences, they sometimes respond by joining the anti-breastfeeding movement.

### Rules and Breastfeeding Do Not Work

It's best to disregard rules altogether for breastfeeding mothers if babies are drinking well from the breast. Most healthcare professionals do not know how to determine this, yet it is the most important skill they can learn. Knowing how to evaluate whether a baby is receiving milk from the breast is easy to learn, yet even some lactation consultants do not have this skill, never mind doctors. We will discuss this more in Chapter 10.

## Who We Are and Why We Wrote This Book

We are Andrea Polokova and Jack Newman and between us is a great deal of experience helping mothers breastfeed. Andrea Polokova is a lactation consultant who has been helping mothers since 2001, and has trained thousands of lactation consultants in Slovakia and the Czech Republic. She frequently speaks at breastfeeding conferences, is an author of a breastfeeding book published in three languages, and has trained lactation consultants in the marginalized Roma communities in Slovakia in cooperation with the Slovak Ministry of Health. Andrea is also a trainer for the Baby-Friendly Hospital Initiative in Slovakia and the Czech Republic.

Dr. Jack Newman is a pediatrician who has helped breastfeeding mothers since 1984. He watched and learned from the nursing staff of a hospital in Umtata in the Republic of South Africa where he worked from 1981 to 1983 (18 months) as chief of pediatrics at that hospital in the Transkei. At the Umtata hospital, many babies and toddlers were very sick from infectious diseases, malnutrition, and kwashiorkor, and a large part of the nurses' work involved re-establishing breastfeeding with babies who were partially or completely formula-fed. Dr. Newman also learned a lot watching his three children being breastfed up to age 4.

Jack Newman and Andrea Polokova have worked together since 2006 and have published a number of articles together, including an eBook called *Breastfeeding: Empowering Parents* and a chapter in a book on clinical pharmacology called *Special Population: Breastfeeding*.

Our goal for this book is to promote dialogue between doctors and mothers, and to help mothers discern if they are getting good advice. We also hope that doctors will read this book so that they can become better breastfeeding supporters and identify myths that might be part of their own practices.

# THE FUNDAMENTALS

# CHAPTER 1

# A Short History of Infant Feeding

Breastfeeding is the biological norm, but even when most mothers breastfed, there have always been some babies not fed at their mothers' breasts. Mothers died, or babies were abandoned. In the Middle Ages, even when there were no "good-enough" substitutes, mothers in some cultures chose not to breastfeed. Tragically, their babies died at shockingly high rates. For example, according to anthropologist Patricia Stuart-McAdam's historical review, mothers in countries such as Iceland, Bohemia, and the Tirol did not breastfeed in the 15th century and 50% of their babies died (Dettwyler & Stuart-McAdam, 1995). Many of those who did not die were stunted in their growth and often were chronically ill throughout their lives.

## Hunter/Gatherer Societies

Learning about hunter/gatherer societies allows us to glimpse life before both agriculture and industrialization. Not surprisingly, these cultures often do not have a written history of themselves, but anthropologists were intensely interested in them during the 20th century, mainly because the way these cultures lived challenged many of the things people believed about relationships, sexuality, and how to feed babies and rear children. We can speculate that breastfeeding must have been near universal as they had no domesticated animals (except for possibly dogs) to provide milk.

Anthropologists who lived amongst such peoples did not see breastfeeding as a topic of particular interest. Margaret Mead, writing about Samoa, for example, briefly mentioned that mothers there breastfed "on demand" but she was more interested and wrote much more about their sexual behavior than about infant feeding. We do know that mothers carried and slept with their babies. They also breastfed for years. Hewlett and colleagues (2014) also found that other mothers sometimes breastfed babies that were not theirs, which may also answer the question about what would happen if a mother did not have enough milk for her baby. According to Hewlett et al. (2014), in 93% of hunter-gather societies, babies are occasionally breastfed by other mothers.

## Wet Nursing

Wet nursing is another form of infant feeding that most Westerners are familiar with. It involves babies being fed at the breast by a mother other than the birth mother. Wet nursing has a long history that we cannot really do justice to in this short space, but we did want to acknowledge its historical importance.

Wet nurses were either paid or forced, in the case of slaves. They were often poor women whose own babies sometimes suffered because they

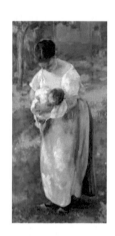

were separated from their mothers or their mothers did not have enough milk for them and the babies they wet nursed. Sometimes the wet nurse lived with the family and sometimes the baby lived in the wet nurse's home. Wet nurses show up in paintings, as below, and in novels, such as Flaubert's *Madame Bovary.*

By the 18th century wet nursing had become relatively common. Jean-Jacques Rousseau strongly recommended that mothers breastfeed their own children and not have other women breastfeed them. By the 19th century, many middle-class families hired wet nurses if they could afford one. However, many babies bonded with their wet nurses, not their biological mothers, as in the painting below (Jean Marie Flouest, 19th century, entitled *Le retour de nourrice avec l'enfant,* The return of the wet nurse with the child). As can be seen in the painting, the child reaches in desperation for the wet nurse and is upset being in his mother's arms.

Unfortunately, many poor women in the 19th century went back to work immediately after birth because they had no other option. Hiring a wet nurse was out of the question. Many of these babies died because they were fed unsafe and inappropriate foods. Another solution seemed necessary.

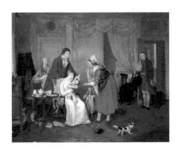

Interestingly, the International Labour Organization (ILO), since 1919, as part of the Peace of Paris, advocated for workers' rights, including the rights of breastfeeding mothers. Workplace support for mothers who are breastfeeding has been a basic provision of maternity protection since the first Maternity Protection Convention (No. 3) in 1919 (International Labour Organization, 2012). A key provision of the Maternity Protection Convention: A woman shall be provided with the right to one or more daily breaks, or a daily reduction of hours of work, so she can breastfeed her child. The break should be a total of one hour, usually divided into two 30 minutes breaks.

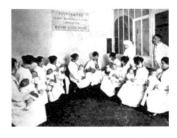

This photo was taken near the end of the 19th century showing women workers at the Louvre in Paris breastfeeding their babies during their break. Allowing women to breastfeed at school or work is common in other parts of the world, as the photos below show.

Unfortunately, allowing mothers to breastfeed during work breaks did not become common practice, so parents started feeding their babies animal milks via a bottle or other feeding device. The milk was not pasteurized and the bottles themselves were not easily cleaned, so the results were tragically predictable. Bacteria, though postulated to exist since the middle-ages, were not thought relevant to disease until the middle of the 19th century. This old drawing shows a "wonderful" invention! No need to even hold the baby.

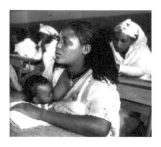
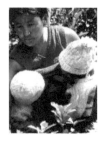
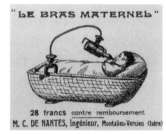

Unscrupulous vendors often diluted or added white substances (lime milk) to "bulk up" the milk. Even without the risk of contaminated milk, straight cow's milk resulted in *healthy looking* "fat" babies who were not really healthy. They could not fight off infections like breastfed babies could. Furthermore, they often became severely anemic as straight cow's milk could cause bleeding from the intestinal tract while containing very little iron. Of course, tuberculosis and other diseases, such as brucellosis, were passed from animals to humans, another source of infant mortality.

## The Advent of Commercial Infant Formula

Lack of breastfeeding happened long before both industrialization and the advent of a commercial infant-feeding industry. However, both dramatically shaped the historical course of breastfeeding. In 1867, Nestle started to advertise a commercial infant formula directly to mothers that was touted as safe and similar to breastmilk. Unfortunately for babies and their mothers, it was neither similar nor safe.

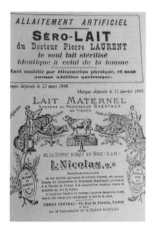

As years went by, more and more "milks for babies," frequently developed by pediatricians with their own special "formulas," became available on the market. This photo of a formula was advertised in 1890s as "the only sterilized milk identical to that of a woman" (word-for-word translation). Identical to a woman's milk? This is incorrect on so many levels. For one thing, breastmilk is *not* sterile. The bacteria in breastmilk are good, not bad, as they help develop an appropriate microbiome in the baby's intestinal tract.

## What Did This "Scientific" Approach Mean for Breastfeeding?

Industrialization and emerging scientific findings undoubtedly improved many aspects of life. Not surprisingly, there were also significant downsides. Eventually this wave of innovation influenced every aspect of life, even childrearing. Formula was promoted as "better than breastmilk." It was measurable and "scientific." It was even called "formula" making it *sound* scientific.

When it came to breastfeeding, physicians and public health nurses told mothers to feed babies fixed amounts according to the clock. "Feed the baby 10 minutes on each breast every 3 hours" was (and still is, unbelievably) typical, though each infant feeding "expert" might have had his (and it was usually "his") own variation. Unfortunately, breastfeeding by the clock has never worked for either mothers or babies. Of course, some mothers ignored the bad advice because it just wasn't practical. Or they may have been too poor to go to see doctors or buy formula. But many other mothers did try to follow the rules. And when babies did not seem satisfied, or were fussy, or spent a lot of time crying, the answer was to supplement. This started the belief that breastfeeding just couldn't work much of the time. The "scientific" approach caused a precipitous decline in breastfeeding. Commercial breastmilk substitutes, heavily marketed as "exactly the same as breastmilk," gradually took over.

## A Bottle-Feeding Society

By the end of the 19th century, a growing middle class could afford doctors and their treatments. Doctors had learned a lot about anatomy but were just learning about the bacterial causes of some diseases, such as typhoid fever, tuberculosis, and cholera. Doctors rejoiced in scientific discoveries. Medicine was leading them into a brave new era of discovery and treatments. However, doctors' lack of knowledge about infectious diseases affected mothers and babies. Mothers did not know that they needed to boil water or sterilize their bottles. As a result, many babies died when they contracted these diseases.

The mentality embedded in physicians' thinking, even in the 21st century, was *that everything will be discovered and cured.* At the beginning of the 20th century, scientists truly believed that their discoveries would result in better ways to feed babies than mothers' own milk. In fact, many doctors still believe that formula is superior to breastmilk.

By the late 19th and early 20th century, formula was the modern way to feed their babies. Breastfeeding was something that only poor women did. By the early 20th century, doctors told new parents how to make infant formula from ingredients available at home: cow's milk, sugar, and water. Each pediatrician had his own method and were thus complicit in breastfeeding's decline. Physicians inserted themselves into a process that had traditionally passed from woman to woman, with the idea that they (physicians) knew best. Even if physicians had wanted to learn about breastfeeding, who could teach them? By the 1960s, few women breastfed, and who would seek feeding information from a mother? Breastfeeding

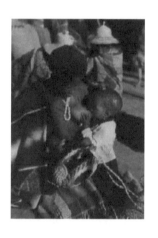

was not the norm in many Western nations, but that was not true in other parts of the world. Take a look at this postcard that I (JN) received from Swaziland in southern Africa.

I have asked many people about what they thought that photo showed. Most answered that breastfeeding in public was not considered a problem, or that breastfeeding a toddler was still common in that area, or other comments along those lines. Interestingly, the caption on the back does not mention breastfeeding at all. Instead, it says, "A woman weaving a basket." Breastfeeding was not the point of this photo. In a culture where breastfeeding is the norm, there is no need to comment on something so widespread. Almost all mothers breastfed, but perhaps only some wove baskets.

The bottle-feeding society has convinced many women that they will not be able breastfeed. They are no longer confident in their bodies' ability to make milk. We received this photo from a pregnant woman who was concerned that her breasts would not to be good for breastfeeding. She had never given birth before, so never breastfed. Why would she be worried? Well, the "why" is what the book is all about.

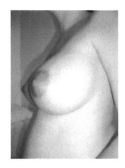

## Formula Companies Keep Up Disinformation

The following pages are from a formula company "information booklet" for parents. They capitalize on parents' number 1 fear: are their babies are getting enough to eat? Want to be sure? The photo tells us the answer: a bottle of formula.

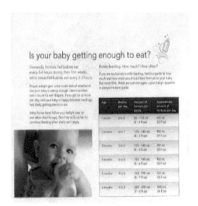
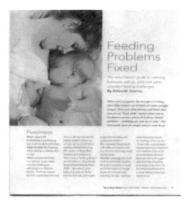

The title of this page "Feeding Problems Fixed" associating feeding problems with breastfeeding. In other words, breastfeeding causes problems and the rest of the booklet gives us the solution. Incidentally, note the unusual position of the mother, a position which is likely to give her pain in the neck. The baby's position is also problematic and is more a bottle-feeding position. (The photo tells us everything we need to know. Try drinking when your head is twisted like that.) These are only two photos of many in this booklet and most like them in other formula company "teaching" booklets, which undermine breastfeeding with both text and photos.

9

## Socialization of Children

Finally, we would like to point out that bottle-feeding socialization begins early and is ubiquitous in toys and books for children. Dolls for children come with bottles so they can practice feeding babies, the "normal way."

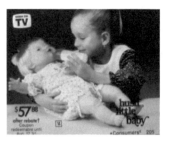

The photos from these children's books are mainly from the 1980s, but remember, that this is the time when many of today's doctors were growing up.

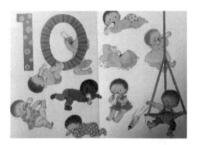
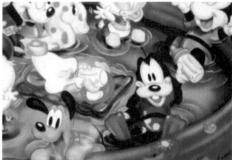
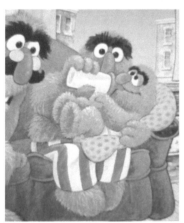
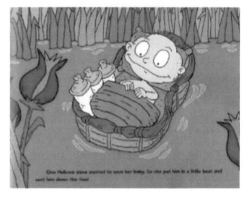

Hundreds of possible photos including the last in the series above, emphasize that even in "ancient Egypt," at the time of the first Passover, babies, including Moses, were all "normally" fed by bottles. What do the following photos say? The left-hand page shows the father and older child feeding the baby a bottle. The child is fascinated, the father feels proud to help out (okay, our interpretation).

And the right-hand page? The mother so exhausted that she fell asleep while breastfeeding the baby and is in danger of dropping the baby. If the mother wakes and leans forward, the rocking chair will likely run over the cat's tail, scaring everyone in the house. It is not exactly a positive depiction of breastfeeding.

# Every day, everywhere,

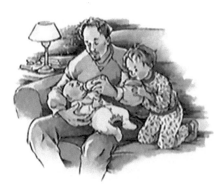 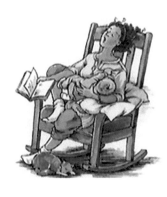

## Conclusion

When all is said and done, it is not surprising that healthcare professionals, like much of the population, just do not "get" breastfeeding. Even some mothers who breastfed successfully do not really understand how breastfeeding works, but they managed it because breastfeeding is *supposed* to work; that's how nature intended it.

## CHAPTER 2

# Medical Education and Breastfeeding

Physicians have many incorrect beliefs about breastfeeding. We will return to this topic throughout this book. Myths may come from their personal experiences of breastfeeding (either as a mother or a partner), or from colleagues, or educational seminars presented by formula companies, or all of the above. For many physicians, however, misinformation starts in medical school.

## What Passes for Medical Education about Breastfeeding

I (JN) received copies of PowerPoint slides from a lecture in 2018 at the University of Toronto teaching first-year medical students about infant feeding. Students see the same presentation every year. One presenter was a pediatrician and professor of pediatrics, the other a nutritionist from University of Toronto's nutrition department. The speakers claim no conflict of interest, but they both work for organizations that accept money from formula companies. Granted, these lecturers may not have personally received any money, but their institutions certainly have. For example, the Hospital for Sick Children accepted money from Mead Johnson Nutrition (a formula company): between $100,000 and $300,000.

In addition, their employer, the University of Toronto received a donation between $100,000 to $999,999 from Abbott Laboratories, a company that also makes infant and toddler formulas. They received the same amount from Bristol-Myers-Squibb Pharmaceutical Group, which, at one point owned Mead Johnson. Nestle, one of the worst offenders undermining breastfeeding with its marketing methods, also donated this amount.

That the speakers plan to describe "the benefits of breastfeeding" speaks volumes about where this lecture is going. Breastfeeding is the *normal physiologic* way of feeding infants, toddlers, and older children. Therefore, one should not be discussing the "benefits" of breastfeeding. Rather, one should be describing the risks to not breastfeeding. It would be like saying "Describe the benefits of good health."

After describing the benefits of breastfeeding, they quickly switch gears. The rest of the presentation is on different types of formula and the indications for each. So, most of this infant feeding lecture for first-year medical students focuses on formula. The lecture also asks attendees to "describe the approach to transitioning to solid food and milk." The slide implies that by 6 months, not only will babies transition to food but also to cows' milk. No mention of breastmilk or breastfeeding. After all, "transitioning" means "moving over to…" Do children really need cow's milk? No, there is nothing magical about it, even if babies never breastfed, as long as they are eating a variety of food in adequate amounts.

Another objective was for learners to "describe the benefits, indications and contraindications of infant formulas and breast milk." This statement strongly suggests equality between the two feeding methods. Since there is only one definite, absolute contraindication to breastfeeding: the rare inborn error of metabolism, galactosemia. One wonders why this is discussed during week 7 of the first year of medical school. What would galactosemia mean to a student 7 weeks into a 4-year program? The student who shared the handout drew an arrow from "otitis media" to what that means: "ear infection."

Another objective was for attendees to "understand the importance of iron and vitamin D supplementation in infancy." What do we learn? That breastmilk is lacking in both. Again, planting doubt on the value of breastfeeding into the minds of these impressionable students. In fact, full-term exclusively breastfeeding babies have adequate iron stores to last at least 6 months assuming that there was not an abnormal loss of blood by baby or mother. As for Vitamin D, some sun exposure will get the baby vitamin D. In Canada, the most common Vitamin D supplement is marketed by a formula company.

They do mention the recommendations of the World Health Organization, which they paraphrased as "exclusive breastfeeding to 6 months, then continued breastfeeding with complementary foods for the next 6 months and beyond." Not exactly. Those are the American Academy of Pediatrics' recommendations, sort of. The WHO recommends continued breastfeeding to 2 years and beyond. Why would the lecturers make this change? Are they afraid to shock students with babies or toddlers breastfeeding to 2 years and beyond? Or maybe they just do not know the real recommendation?

Another slide describes the contraindications to breastmilk. These include galactosemia, but what they described was not quite true. It is only true for the full spectrum, not the partial (Duarte) version, though not all experts agree that breastfeeding is safe even with the Duarte variation. Next is untreated tuberculosis. Well, the answer is to start treatment of both mother and baby (see Chapter 19). They then list HIV, but HIV is no longer considered a contraindication for breastfeeding. The World Health Organization now recommends breastfeeding if a mother is HIV+ and being treated during the pregnancy, and after the baby is born, and then the baby is treated from birth.

The next contraindication was illegal drug use. Well, this is controversial. We believe that it is better to encourage new mothers to breastfeed and get them off narcotics rather that proscribe breastfeeding (note that cannabis was legal in Canada at the time of this lecture).

Next on the list of contraindications was simply "medication": that any medication taken by the mother contraindicates breastfeeding. This is clearly not true, though many physicians act as if it were. In fact, most medications are compatible with breastfeeding (see Chapter 20). The next line asks the student to check with the Mother Risk Clinic at the hospital. (The only problem is that the Mother Risk Clinic does not exist anymore.)

That is the end of the slides that "discuss breastfeeding." A total of 5 slides (out of 54), including one on contraindications to breastfeeding. Most of the "breastfeeding" slides give incorrect, dubious, or biased information. Perhaps breastfeeding was explained in more detail during the lecture itself but given the number of slides for a 1-hour lecture, this seems unlikely.

The first 5 slides are now followed by *12* slides on formula-feeding. Oddly, the students learn that they will get a taste test of various formulas, the purpose of which is not clear, followed by a discussion of the reasons for using different formulas. For the healthy full-term baby, they recommend regular cows'-milk-based formula. For gastroesophageal reflux, there is special anti-reflux formula. For babies of vegan parents, there is soy formula, etc. These slides are followed by multiple slides on feeding babies food that can only be questioned as "old fashioned," instilling fear of iron deficiency and bottle caries (see Chapter 21).

This example is not uncommon. I (JN) recently received a link for a medical continuing education course entitled, "Infant nutrition: Balancing the building blocks of brain development and immune support." Here is how they described the course.

The first months and early years of life set the stage for lifelong development. It is within those first 3 to 5 years that the greatest percentage of an infant's brain growth occurs. During this significant time, it's important to understand the role of nutrition in brain development and immune support as a child grows.

It sounds good, doesn't it? The entire course is on formula and is, not surprisingly, funded by Mead Johnson, a formula company (MD BriefCase, 2021).

A 2011 study of 103 pediatric program directors found that pediatric residents received 9 hours of breastfeeding training over 3 years, or 3 hours per year (Osband, Altman, Patrick, & Edwards, 2011). In addition, while 67% to 75% provided breastfeeding rooms or breast pumps, only 10 programs had an official policy to accommodate breastfeeding pediatric residents. A more recent study found that OB residents received more breastfeeding education than pediatric or family medicine residents, but that 75% of respondents cited barriers to receiving this education (Lien & Shattuck, 2017).

## Common Myths that Health Professionals Believe

Given this lack of evidence-based and accurate education, it should not surprise anyone that physicians have many mistaken ideas about breastfeeding. We will discuss a few myths now, but subsequent chapters will cover other topics in depth.

### There Is No Milk in The First Few Days

Nonsense! Milk starts accumulating in the breast from about 16 weeks of pregnancy. This myth results in babies receiving bottles of formula sometimes from the very first feeding after birth, even in 2022. Mothers can express milk even before the baby is born. We recommend that mothers whose babies are at risk for being supplemented from birth, such as when the mother has diabetes, start expressing milk before the baby is born (see Chapter 8).

### Okay, There Might Be Milk in The First Few Days, But It's Not Enough

Ridiculous. The amount of milk babies gets depends on how well they latch on to the breast. Strong hint: if the mother has nipple pain, the baby is *not* latched on well. Nipple pain is never normal but should be a "call to action" for the hospital staff. It's better to fix problems soon after birth rather than waiting 3 weeks or even longer, when we usually see mothers and babies.

### Bottle-Feeding Breastmilk and Breastfeeding Are the Same

Feeding a baby by bottle (even with breastmilk) and the baby feeding at the breast are not the same. Many babies who are frequently bottle-fed eventually refuse the breast. When doctors think they are the same, they miss the bigger picture. Breastfeeding is a close, intimate, physical, and emotional relationship between the mother and baby that cannot be duplicated even by bottle-feeding breastmilk. Of course, mothers can bond with their babies if they're bottle-feeding. In fact, we want them to. Developing a close relationship with the baby is important no matter how the baby is fed, but breastfeeding supports a close physical and emotional relationship between mother and baby. The baby is attached to this very sensitive part of the mother's body and that is why it is important that breastfeeding not hurt.

Some argue that normal labor and birth are very painful. Yes, but when the baby is born, the pain should go away. How wonderful an association! Painful breastfeeding can go away on its own, but not for many days or weeks, and it does not *always* go away. Thus, it is not the same as giving birth. The pain of breastfeeding may last for weeks or months if the mother does not get good help.

### Babies Do Not Gain Weight Because Their Mothers' Milk Is "Thin" and Does Not Contain Enough Fat or Calories

Fat content of breastmilk varies from mother to mother, but it increases as a breastfeed continues in all mothers. Thus, if babies are not drinking well, or the feedings are limited, say, to 10 minutes/side, babies may not gain well. Not because of "thin" milk but because of poor advice. Interestingly, fat content also increases after 12 months of breastfeeding (Mandel, Lubetzky, Dollberg, Barak, & Mimouni, 2005).

## Not Enough Milk

Unfortunately, many health professionals believe that mothers probably cannot make enough milk for their babies. They might say, "Well, nothing in biology works all the time. Some mothers just do not produce enough milk." It is true that some mothers cannot produce all that their babies need, but many mothers who are told to supplement probably didn't need to. In her novel *The Group*, first published in 1963, Mary McCarthy has a long chapter in which she discusses how the mothers, the principal characters in the novel, ended up "failing at breastfeeding." Just one quote will speak volumes:

> "Have you got a watch?" Norine asked, yawning. Priss told her the time. "Are you nursing?" she asked, stealing an envious look at Norine's massive breasts. "My milk ran out," said Norine. "So did mine!" cried Priss. "As soon as I left the hospital. How long did

*you* nurse?" "Four weeks. Then Freddy slept with the girl we had looking after Ichabod, and my milk went on strike." Priss gulped; the story she had been about to relate, of how her milk had run out as soon as they gave Stephen a supplementary bottle, was hastily vetoed on her lips.

I (JN) remember liking the book but was shocked how doctors undermined one of the main character's breastfeeding. The husband of one character was a pediatrician who verbally supported her breastfeeding while undermining it with poor advice. Another quote from *The Group*:

> Mrs. Harshorn glanced at her daughter and lowered her voice. "Just fancy little Priss being the first of your set to do it, Polly. She's so flat she's never had to wear a brassière. But Sloan says it's not the size that counts. I do hope he's right. The miracle of the loaves and fishes, *I* call it. All the other babies in the nursery are on bottles. The nurses prefer it that way. I'm inclined to agree with them. Doctors are all theory. Nurses see the facts." She swallowed her martini in a single draft, like medicine; this was the style among advanced society women of her age. She wiped her lips and refused a "dividend" from the silver shaker. "Which way progress, Polly?" she demanded, in a slightly louder voice, shaking her white bobbed locks. "The bottle was the war-cry of my generation. Linda was bottle-fed. And you can't imagine the difference. For us, the bottle spelled the end of colic, and your frantic husband walking the baby all night. We swore by the bottle, we of the avant-grade. My mother-in-law was horripilated. And now, I confess, Polly, I'm horripilated myself."

## How Things Have **Not** Changed!

I'd (JN) like to close this chapter by sharing an anecdote from my (JN) training at the University of Toronto. In 1969, we had a 1-hour on infant feeding in our medical school's fourth and final year. The pediatrician stood in front of the class and said, "Breast is best because it always comes at the right temperature and comes in such cute containers" (I am not joking, but this was another era and another way of thinking).

He then continued the lecture with "Now I will discuss infant formula" and the whole rest of the 1-hour lecture was devoted to how to make formula from whole milk, water, and sugar (often in the form of corn syrup, which was supposed to duplicate breastmilk). We doubt that pediatricians really thought that the formula would truly duplicate breastmilk, but nevertheless, he and most other pediatricians obviously believed *it did not really matter.* Milk was milk and that was that.

A note on the second quote from *The Group.* Did bottle feeding really end "colic"? No, because it is our strong belief that "colic" does not occur in exclusively breastfed babies. So called "colic" is almost always due to babies just wanting more milk, even if they are gaining very well. (See Chapter 14.)

# CHAPTER 3

# Is Formula the Same as Breastmilk?

This question is at the heart of healthcare providers' attitudes about breast-feeding. It's reflected in their education, and it is reflected in their motivation, or lack of motivation, for educating themselves about breastfeeding. Think about it from the physicians' standpoint. If you believe that formula is "just as good," why would you bother to support breastfeeding or try to help a mother get over her difficulties? As we've described previously, at the first sign of trouble, without skills to solve breastfeeding problems, formula seems a viable alternative.

Formula company marketing wants us to believe that formula-feeding is normal, a personal choice, and that it is almost as good as breastmilk. Outrageously, the under-the-breath message is that formula is *better* than breastfeeding because it is safer and more reliable. Formula companies deliver this message to parents and the health professionals who counsel them. If you think breastfeeding usually fails, formula is appealing.

Unfortunately, the general population often shares this view. In our early days at the breastfeeding clinic, mothers not infrequently came with their own mothers (and still do). We asked the grandmothers if they had breastfed their children. Many said, "I wanted to breastfeed, but the 'baby doctor' told me that formula was better."

During the late 1980s, when we saw a mother, baby, and grandmother, the new mothers were usually born in the late 1950s and 1960s, an era when breastfeeding initiation was at its nadir: 20% to 25% of mothers initiated breastfeeding. A few mothers managed to breastfeed, but they were the exceptions.

## "New and Improved"

Formula has come a long way since its milk-and-corn-syrup days. Formula companies spend millions to study breastmilk and identify components, which means that they continually add things to their products, thus admitting their formulas are less-than-good copies of breastmilk. The real issue is that breastfeeding is much more than the sum of its parts. Ingredients in breastmilk interact with each other, augmenting the function of some constituents while inhibiting the function of others. Formula cannot duplicate these interactions regardless of added new ingredients. Nevertheless, companies persist because new added ingredients are the basis of new advertising. You cannot keep flogging the same advertising year after year, as the effect of such advertising diminishes with repetition. Below is a partial list of things formula "scientists" have added to infant formula over the past couple of decades to try to make it "more like breastmilk."

### Long-Chain Polyunsaturated Fats (LC-PUFAs)

LC-PUFAs were added to formula because they are essential for brain and vision development. DHA (docosahexaenoic acid), an Omega-3 fatty acid, and ARA (arachidonic acid), an Omega-6 fatty acid are the LC-PUFAs added to formula. Ads promised that these formulas would help babies see better and make them smarter. These brands were more expensive, but parents gladly paid (if they could afford it, and even if they could not afford it) because, of course, they wanted their babies to be smart. Unfortunately, these special formulas did not live up the hype. They did not increase babies' intelligence nor was their vision better according to a recent Cochrane review (Jasani, Simmer, Patole, & Rao, 2017). Nevertheless, advertising still sells lots of formula. Remember that the ingredients in breastmilk do not act in isolation; they interact with other components and often this interaction does not occur if all the ingredients involved in the interaction are not in the formula.

## Lowered Protein Content

Formula has always had more protein than babies need. Most formulas are made with cows' milk. Baby cows need a lot of protein, but human infants do not. Too much protein increases the risk of childhood and adult obesity, as well as increasing the risk of chronic high blood pressure (Oropeza et al., 2018; Patro-Golab et al., 2016). In response to these findings, lower-protein formulas have been developed. This is good news for infants who need to rely on formula, but the levels are still too high. Why are they still too high?

Protein levels are not just about the concentration of protein in formula. Lactoferrin comprises most of the protein in breastmilk (60% to 65% of the total). This protein is not bioavailable meaning it is *not absorbed from the intestinal tract.* Another 6% or so of the protein is made up of the antibodies in breastmilk, which the baby also does not absorb, and which remains in the intestine. This means that the bioavailable protein in breastmilk is much lower than even the "lower" amounts now in formulas. Sadly, instead of saying "sorry, we didn't know," formula manufacturers chose to avoid the bad optics and have adopted the lowered protein concentration as a marketing stratagem to excitedly market how wonderful the new and improved formulas are.

## Nucleotides

Nucleotides were a big deal in the 1990s and are one of many immune ingredients in breastmilk, so formula companies added them to their products. Unfortunately, nucleotides *in formulas* don't do much of anything. Nucleotides are *part* of a system of immune components, not simply one ingredient acting on its own. If you only add nucleotides, or any single ingredient, or even a few ingredients of the immune system of breastfeeding, you do not get the effect of the full immune system.

Nucleotides have always been in breastmilk. I (JN) recall a meeting at the Hospital for Sick Children (Toronto) where one of the pediatricians, a specialist in infant nutrition, spoke highly of the importance of adding nucleotides to formula. A pediatrician in the audience questioned whether nucleotides were really so important in formula. The specialist in infant nutrition stated that they were definitely important, implying it was a revolutionary change. If that were true, why do we never hear about nucleotides in formula now? Basically, because the revolution was a bust. Nucleotides added to formula do not an immune system make.

## Oligosaccharides

Oligosaccharides are the much-vaunted prebiotics that were added to formulas in the last two decades. Formula companies made a big deal about adding this ingredient. They've *always* been in breastmilk.

## Probiotics

Probiotics are microorganisms added to formulas supposedly to encourage the growth of good bacteria in the baby's gut. Scientists have learned that an appropriate gut flora is critical for long-term health. Formula companies have now added probiotics to create healthy gut flora. Probiotics received so much hype that even breastfeeding mothers have been buying them to give to their babies. Not surprisingly, breastmilk has *always* contained probiotics, which promotes the growth of desirable bacteria in the baby's gut. And not to overstate the point but adding probiotics to formula does not an immune system make.

## Milk Fat Globules

Milk fat globules were added to formulas. These aid in maturation in the function and structure of the gut and the provision of nutrients (Lee et al., 2018). These have always been in breastmilk.

## Formulas for Specific Problems

In addition to adding ingredients, formula companies make products to address any infant malady from spitting up to allergy. Most of this is strictly marketing hype. These special formulas are expensive and completely unnecessary (such as toddler milks, even up to ages 3 to 5 years). Unfortunately, formula companies are brilliant at marketing, and they prey on parents' fears. For that matter, they also prey on physicians' fears that breastfeeding will fail, and babies will starve. If there are problems, better to be "safe" than sorry.

## What Formula Lacks

Even with billions spent on breastmilk research, even with special ingredients added, formula will *never* be equal to breastmilk because breastmilk is living tissue, with a complex web of components that interact with each other in different ways under difference circumstances. Interestingly, for all the hype about adding ingredients to make formula "like breastmilk," there are dozens of components of breastmilk that were identified decades ago but have never been added to formula. Here are a few examples.

### HAMLET (Human Alpha-lactalbumin Made Lethal to Tumor cells)

This compound, always present in breastmilk, causes tumor cells to "commit suicide" (apoptosis; (Gustafsson et al., 2005).

### Epidermal Growth Factor

Epidermal growth factor is important for the development, maturation, and protection of the intestinal mucosa (lining). Epidermal growth factor protects the baby's gut from the devastating damage that can be caused by necrotizing enterocolitis, which occurs primarily in premature babies (Dvorak, 2010).

### Neuronal Growth Factor

Neuronal growth factor plays a key role in neuroprotection and developmental maturity (Sanchez-Infantes et al., 2018).

### Cytokines

Various cytokines (compounds that vary the immune response) and cytokine inhibitors (Dawod & Marshall, 2019). Cytokines work together with other cytokines and components of breastmilk: some cytokines inhibit the actions of other compounds/factors, while augmenting the actions of others.

Some switch sides by inhibiting actions under certain circumstances and augmenting under others. Considerable evidence confirms the importance of all these factors and their interactions in the health of the growing baby and child. Nature rarely does something for nothing.

Furthermore, components in breastmilk can vary quite widely. In this study, the authors found that they needed to measure the amount of iron, zinc, and copper in the mother's milk on 11 consecutive days for iron, three consecutive days for zinc, and 10 for copper to be 95% confident that the measures were correct (Dhonukshe-Rutten et al., 2005). In other words, the amounts varied day to day. It is generally easy to measure to measure iron, zinc, and copper and this study suggests that it may be much more difficult to measure the "true" amounts of proteins or other biological compounds in the breastmilk. Variation of breastmilk components seems to be the rule rather than the exception.

How do formula manufacturers deal with this problem? How much should they add to their formulas if they decide to add, for example, HAMLET to their milks? Could lactoferrin in formula be turned into HAMLET? To make HAMLET, the liquid in the stomach needs to be acidic (low pH), as it is in the breastfed baby. Unfortunately, the liquid in the stomach of the formula-fed baby likely has too high a pH to make HAMLET.

Here's another example. The amount of iron in formulas is often much greater than it is in breastmilk. Iron was added to formula to prevent iron-deficiency anemia found in exclusively formula-fed babies. This was a particular problem in lower-economic communities, whose families might find it difficult to provide iron-rich foods for their babies, such as meat, fish, or poultry.

However, is more always better? Can there be too much iron in formula? Too much iron can be a problem because many harmful bacteria thrive on iron, may multiply to worrisome numbers, and cause illness in the baby. Quinn (2014) addresses this issue. The amount of iron in breastmilk is just right. Too much iron in formula supports the growth of pathogenic bacteria in the baby's gut. If the baby is exclusively breastfed until the recommended 6 months, and the baby starts eating iron-rich food when their immune system is more mature, they are more likely to be able to fight off the pathogenic bacteria, aided by continued breastfeeding.

## Breastmilk Also Varies by Time of Day

Breastmilk also differs from formula in that it changes over the course of a day, and it varies by day or nighttime. This area of study is known as "chrononutrition" (Hahn-Holbrook, Saxbe, Bixby, Steele, & Glynn, 2019). Circadian rhythms govern breastmilk (daily cycles of sleep and waking). Interestingly, pumped "daytime" milk at night may interfere with babies' sleep patterns, as Hahn-Holbrook et al. note.

> Expressed milk is not necessarily circadian-matched…and may disrupt infants' developing circadian rhythms, potentially contributing to sleep problems and decreased physiological attunement with their mothers and environments (p. 936).

Mothers and physicians may interpret these findings to mean that breastmilk can be given at the "wrong time." If this is a concern, remember that infant formulas have *no circadian rhythm;* it is always the same regardless of the time of the day, month, or year.

## Breastmilk Varies by the Child's Age

We described chrononutrition in the previous section because it's important and it's a great example of something that most health professionals don't know about. Something we've known about for a longer time is that breastmilk varies depending on infant's age. Breastmilk for a newborn differs from that of breastmilk for an older baby. Consider this question I (JN) received from a health professional. It made me scratch my head.

> I had a call today from a woman whose sister, who is a drug user, delivered a baby today. The baby remains in hospital and is being treated for drug withdrawal. The mother has abandoned the infant and the baby will be cared for by an aunt. My question is this: the caregiver wants to breastfeed this newborn as she is still nursing her own 11-month-old. Is

her milk appropriate for this infant or should the baby be supplemented with formula as well?

Truly, I did not know how to address this at first. Formula *never* changes regardless of age. Why is that more acceptable for the baby than breastmilk? We can reasonably ask the question: How old was the calf whose mother "donated" the milk that was made into formula?

## Commercial Infant Formula and the Microbiome

A final issue we'd like to describe is something called the baby's gut microbiome. The microbiome is the balance of good and bad bacteria in the baby's gut. The microbiome has important implications for long-term health. Not surprisingly, how a baby is fed influences the balance of good and bad bacteria (Sim et al., 2013). Breastfed and formula-fed babies have very different bacteria in their intestines and elsewhere. Breastmilk promotes a healthy microbiome because of its many immune properties, which suppress the growth of undesirable bacteria. The microbiome may affect the child's:

- Development including neurological, motor, social, and cognitive development (Clarke, O'Mahony, Dinan, & Cryan, 2014; Codagnone, Stanton, O'Mahony, Dinan, & Cryan, 2019)

- Immune function and protection against pathogens (Johnson & Versalovic, 2012)

- Digestive function (Johnson & Versalovic, 2012)

- And possibly many other systems.

The microbiome seems key to understanding many adult health problems. As Clarke and colleagues (2014) suggest.

We are only beginning to appreciate the potential health benefits that could be accrued from this venture across diagnostic, preventative, and treatment realms. We look forward with great anticipation to this transformed appreciation of how our microbial wealth during early life primes for health in adulthood (p. 817).

Many factors influence the gut microbiome: type of birth, antibiotics the mother or baby receive, who handles the baby first, and feeding method.

This chapter focuses on how breastmilk differs from formula. Breastmilk is alive with immune factors that seed a healthy gut microbiome, and it influences long-term health, long after breastfeeding has ended. A manufactured product can never do this, especially breastmilk that the baby drinks directly from the breast. Sugar and iron in formula may lead to an overgrowth of harmful bacteria and other organisms in the gut, increasing the risk of a wide range of health problems.

## Do Studies Show Any Real Difference?

People who oppose breastfeeding claim that research shows no real difference in health outcomes for babies breastfed and those formula fed, insisting that studies that *do* show better health outcomes for the breastfed babies are not well done. For example, some claim that studies showing better outcomes for the mothers and their breastfed babies are not valid unless they are randomized controlled trials. This design is considered the "gold standard" for testing things like whether a medication works, for example. This design requires random assignment to those who receive the medication or those who receive a placebo, and the results are compared. However, it would be highly unethical to assign some mothers to breastfeeding and some to formula-feeding, so researchers need to use other research designs. Does lack of randomized trial mean that breastfeeding studies are flawed? Of course not. Every type of study design has strengths and weaknesses. Researchers need to use a design that is appropriate to the issue being studied and ethical concerns.

A problem in older studies was inconsistent definitions of breastfeeding. For example, exclusive breastfeeding differs physiologically from mixed breastfeeding and formula-feeding, and they are both different even from exclusive breastmilk feeding by bottle. But if mothers from those three groups are combined into one "breastfeeding" group, it will obscure any differences between breastfeeding and formula-feeding groups.

Another methodological issue is conflating breastfeeding with breastmilk feeding. Breastfeeding (i.e., feeding at the breast) differs physiologically from feeding breastmilk by bottle. This can influence, for example, findings about whether breastfeeding prevents ear infection (otitis media). The anti-breastfeeding camp claims that breastfeeding does not prevent ear infection, but if breastfed and breastmilk-fed babies are grouped together, the differences may wash out. A study of 813 women found that breastfeeding was more likely to prevent otitis media than breastmilk in a bottle (Boone, Geraghty, & Keim, 2016). These findings are consistent with earlier results indicating that bottles themselves, even when they contain breastmilk, may predispose infants to otitis media because of intraoral negative pressure to the middle ear (C. E. Brown & Magnuson, 2000).

Even when there are good studies, people tend to be guided by their own experiences. If a health professional's children were not breastfed, and their children are "okay," they may be less likely to promote breastfeeding or encourage new mothers to breastfeed. Many mothers have told us that that their doctor basically stated that there are no advantages to breastfeeding and that they didn't offer to help with breastfeeding difficulties or refer to someone who could help.

## Conclusion

Human milk is the appropriate food for infants and, with added food, for toddlers. Nothing compares to it. In this chapter, we've compared some aspects of breastfeeding, breastmilk, and formula and hope you are convinced that breastmilk and feeding at the breast cannot be duplicated in a laboratory. As we say that, we have separated milk from the act of feeding. As amazing as milk is, it is only one part of the equation. Breastfeeding is much more than breastmilk; it's a relationship, a topic we will revisit in subsequent chapters.

# CHAPTER 4

# The Right to Breastfeed

Women have the right to breastfeed their babies. Unfortunately, women's rights may be circumvented by poorly informed health professionals, judges, and even child protective agents. Even when well-meaning, these professionals have the potential to cause great harm.

## System Failures Force Mothers to Use Formula

Mothers have often trusted the healthcare system to help them breastfeed. Instead of helping mothers make breastfeeding work, the healthcare system often compels mothers to use formula. The mothers frequently feel like they "failed," when it's more accurate to say that *they were failed*. Mothers blame themselves when breastfeeding goes awry, not the hospital practices around labor, birth, and postpartum that undermined them. We see this pattern very often in our clinic. Babies receive a bottle of formula for a first feed because "there is no milk in the first few days," even in teaching hospitals. Unfortunately, mothers often respond by turning against breastfeeding rather than the systems that undermined their breastfeeding. They want to prevent others from having similar experiences.

### Failure to Help with Medical Problems

Mothers may also be told that they should stop breastfeeding for medical reasons, but they might have continued breastfeeding if they had the correct information. In most cases, they did not need to stop. Here are a few examples of when this might occur.

#### Cleft Palate

Cleft palate is one situation where mothers are told that they cannot breastfeed and should not bother trying. True, many babies with cleft palate do not seem to be able latch on to the breast, *but some can.* One thing is certain, however. If mothers do not even try, breastfeeding will not work. At the very least, mothers should be allowed to see if their babies can breastfeed.

### Breast-Reduction Surgery

Mothers who have had breast-reduction surgery are routinely told to not breastfeed, yet so much depends on the type of surgery they had. Many are told something along the lines of "chances of breastfeeding are 50%," whatever that means. Some can produce all the milk their babies need while others may not be able to bring in a full supply. However, even when mothers do not have a full supply, they can still feed their babies with donor milk or formula using a lactation aid at the breast.

Supplementing at the breast is important because breastfeeding is so much more than breast milk. It is a close, intimate relationship between two people who love each other. The value of that relationship is not measured by how much breast milk the mother can produce. Health professionals need to see breastfeeding as a relationship that should be maintained even if mothers cannot produce all the milk their babies require. Also, babies well latched on, almost always receive more from the breast than a pump can extract. If we want to maximize the amount of milk babies get from their mothers, feeding at the breast is important.

In addition, some mothers who have had breast-reduction surgery are able to produce enough milk. We have worked with a few mothers who, with help, were able to exclusively breastfeed for 6 months and then continue breastfeeding along with complementary food. In one case, a mother was able to breastfeed twins exclusively for 6 months and then continued with added food. True, she needed domperidone to help her breastfeed the twins exclusively, but what exactly is wrong with that?

### Medications

Most medications are compatible with breastfeeding, but too many mothers are told they must interrupt or stop breastfeeding to take medication. Some medications are contraindicated while breastfeeding, but it's a relatively small number. In many cases, acceptable alternatives are available. See Chapter 20 for more specific information.

## Breastfeeding and Legal Issues

Even when things are going well, mothers are being told to stop breastfeeding altogether for specious psychological reasons, such as that breastfeeding will make their child be "overdependent." Worse still is that some mental health professionals believe that breastfeeding is "sexual," and that breastfeeding past a few weeks is sexual abuse. This claim is bizarre, but more than a few people believe it. Part of their reasoning is that the "true" function of breasts is sexual and that breasts are not for feeding babies, especially not toddlers. That argument doesn't hold up to scrutiny. Many parts of our bodies have more than one function. The mouth, for example, is for eating, but it is also for whistling, playing the oboe, and kissing.

One child psychiatrist in France is frequently cited in the media. In an interview to a widely read Belgian newspaper, he stated, "One does not share the breast: to extend breastfeeding past 7 months is without doubt sexual abuse" (*Le Soir*, November 29, 2003). Amazingly, the media seeks him out for advice on infant psychiatry. The mind boggles. If you believe your child needs to see a psychiatrist, avoid this one.

### Custody Cases

Judges can also interfere with women's right to breastfeed when adjudicating access and custody cases. Frequently, these judges do not include the needs of the breastfed baby or toddler in their decisions, even though the guiding principle in these cases is, supposedly, the best interests of the child. Both parents' needs can be accommodated in terms of spending time with babies. Unfortunately, judges often treat breastfeeding babies and toddlers the same as their formula-feeding counterparts. They do not understand why a non-breastfeeding parent cannot just "give a bottle." Women judges are not necessarily more sympathetic towards mothers. In fact, they can often be less so.

Nursing toddlers can also be forced to do overnight visits with the non-breastfeeding parent. Whether one agrees or not, breastfeeding babies and toddlers derive security, comfort, and yes, love, from breastfeeding. This is also true for babies, but appears more obvious in breastfeeding toddlers, who may have an even harder time leaving their mothers for overnight visits. The last feedings a toddler will generally give up are those in the night. Yet, in custody cases, the non-breastfeeding parent often insists on having the child at night. What is so wonderful about custody of the child at night, when presumably the child is sleeping most of the time? Yes, the picture of parents looking at their sleeping babies with tenderness and tears of joy is lovely. Except the true picture is rarely like that. Most breastfeeding toddlers will not take a bottle, and the non-breastfeeding parent has no way to calm the child in the night. A cup of milk will not work; it's the breast the baby or toddler wants, not necessarily the milk. This can be a horrible experience for everyone involved.

One of our students had her ex-partner bring the toddler back in the middle of the night because the child would not settle after walking up and down the hall, or with the bottle, or with food. I (JN) have received similar emails from many others. Judges do not seem to understand the problem. Too often the breastfeeding mother is accused of deliberately continuing to breastfeed to prevent the father from having his right to access. Nothing is impossible in the custody battle between the parents, but if children do not want to breastfeed, mothers cannot force them. As mentioned previously, breastfeeding is not just about nutrition, a notion that is obviously foreign to so many people, including judges.

## Child-Protection Cases

In many areas, child protective services are a huge problem. Instead of helping mothers continue to breastfeed, CPS tell mothers to, "Stop breast-feeding, give formula, or we will apprehend your child." These workers just do not understand that help is possible. The most recent case I (JN) saw was that of a 6-month-old baby who was not gaining weight well. The pediatrician insisted that the baby receive formula. When the mother refused, he called child protection services. I saw the mother and baby at our clinic and realized that the best, easiest way to deal with the situation was to have the mother add food (why did the pediatrician not consider this for a 6-month-old baby?) and to feed the baby on both breasts at a feeding. For some strange reason, a lactation consultant told her to feed on one breast only at each feeding, which is not a good idea (actually, this is a common recommendation, for reasons beyond our ken). After making these changes, the baby started to gain weight well, but the child protection services were unhappy. The mother did not listen to them—the mother was supposed to give formula. So, they apprehended the baby anyway, even though the baby started to gain weight well based on our approach. They showed her, didn't they? It is not irrelevant that the mother is Indigenous. At least in our community, child protection services have a lower threshold for taking children away from Indigenous parents.

I met another Indigenous mother whose first child was taken by the Child Protective Services because the child was abused by the father. The mother became pregnant again with a different father (she was no longer with the father of the first child). At birth, the child was immediately apprehended by the Child Protection Services. There was no evidence that the mother's new partner was abusing drugs, or was aggressive, or physically abusive. Nothing at all, but she lost the baby. She came to our clinic because the parents got the baby back after several months, and she wanted to relactate. I am sure that this baby would not have been apprehended if the parents were not Indigenous.

## Conclusion

These issues are just a few of dozens of situations when mothers are unnecessarily told, or even *forced* to stop breastfeeding. And if we see dozens, nay hundreds, every year, how many more are told to stop? Most of the time, the problems could have been prevented or treated without using formula or stopping breastfeeding. But in many cases, the mothers do not get the help they need.

If we went through all the situations we hear about daily—situations when mothers do not have the right to breastfeed even though they made an informed decision to do so—we would be writing something longer than *War and Peace.* We are not saying that breastfeeding will always work, even with the best of help, but a lot more mothers and babies could be successful. Speaking of Rights, according to the United Nations Children's Fund, breastfeeding is the *child's right* too.

Every infant and child have the *right* to good nutrition according to the *Convention on the Rights of the Child* (UNICEF, 1989).

# THE POSTPARTUM PERIOD

# CHAPTER 5

# Is Breastfeeding Risky?

In the early 1980s, a *Time Magazine* article identified breastfeeding as "a risky behavior." The article's focus was breastfeeding with HIV and featured an African woman breastfeeding on the cover. At the time, health officials told HIV+ women not to breastfeed as they could infect their babies. However, they soon realized that they needed a more nuanced approach, one that accounted for the *risks* of feeding their babies formula, which in resource-poor areas were very significant. I (JN) worked from 1981 to 1983 as a pediatrician in the Transkei, a part of South Africa, where formula-fed babies died almost daily. Many mothers were poor, so poor that it would be difficult for North Americans to understand. Formula was often diluted with polluted water, the only water available, or even *overdiluted* to save money. In such circumstances, is it better to avoid breastfeeding when the risk of infant death from formula-feeding was a real possibility? I wrote *Time* a letter to the editor, but it was not published.

Putting aside the issue of HIV, the idea of "breastfeeding as dangerous stuck." Many, including many health professionals, believe that breastfeeding is intrinsically risky, whereas formula-feeding is intrinsically safe. Many pediatricians think this too. Why else would we get so many questions about whether medication is safe while breastfeeding? For example, "Can I take collagen when breastfeeding"? Collagen is a normal part of the body, found almost everywhere in the body: in bone, muscle, liver, heart, and in many foods we eat. Of course, it's safe to take, but mothers and healthcare professionals still worry especially when product inserts say, "not recommended if you are breastfeeding"? People have the same reaction to prescribed medications. If doctors do not know whether a medication is compatible with breastfeeding, and most medications are, in fact, compatible, breastfeeding mothers are nevertheless told, "better not breastfeed and play it safe." (More on medications in Chapter 20.)

Finally, people fear the experience of breastfeeding itself: they have heard of breastfeeding causing agonizingly sore nipples, and mastitis, and even breast abscess. They may have heard many horror stories from friends. Mothers have heard that breastfeeding is not good for families, that breastfed babies never sleep and always demand to feed. Then there is the concern that if babies breastfeed for "too long," they will be too clingy, and may even have identity problems, especially boys.

## The Media and Breastfeeding

Science writers and reporters, in general, are no better educated about breastfeeding than health professionals. Why would they be? They learn about breastfeeding from the same health professionals who do not know anything about it. In addition, the media seems to relish horror stories of breastfed babies becoming dehydrated, seriously ill, or even dying. People blame breastfeeding rather than the inept helpers who did not spot the problems that could have been fixed easily if addressed in the first few days of the baby's life.

We are not trying to say that breastfeeding is always trouble free. A small minority of mothers truly cannot produce enough milk, but it is healthcare professionals' job to educate themselves, mothers, and their partners to identify and prevent possible problems. Unfortunately, it's an uphill battle; the healthcare system intrinsically undermines breastfeeding.

### "Overselling Breastfeeding"

Dr. Courtney Jung, a Canadian professor at the University of Toronto, published an opinion piece in the *New York Times* entitled, Overselling Breastfeeding (Jung, 2015, Oct 16). She is not a professor of nutrition, mind you, but a professor of political science. Dr. Jung stated that during her pregnancy, everyone told her how important breastfeeding was. That irritated her. Why? Was she irritated by people telling her she should be eating for two now that she was pregnant? Furthermore, her prenatal teacher would not discuss "formula-feeding because it was not allowed by hospital regulations." What is wrong with the prenatal teacher not discussing for-mula-feeding? The directions are on the tin. You mix the formula with water and feed the baby until the baby is full. Incidentally, the WHO/UNICEF Baby-Friendly Hospital Initiative states that mothers who *choose* artifi-cial feeding should receive *individual* teaching, not in front of the entire prenatal class. Dr. Jung's assertion about the teacher not being allowed to talk about formula is simply not true. Talking about artificial feeding in front of the entire class would suggest equivalency of breastfeeding and formula-feeding.

So, before Dr. Jung gave birth, she was "pretty fed up," though she does not specify why or with what. Fair enough, many pregnant women have mixed feelings about becoming mothers, and the feelings are not always beautiful ones. They might be worried about birth, but they are not generally "fed up" about breastfeeding before the baby is even born. Most accept the notion that breastfeeding is a good thing, and as Dr. Jung herself writes, 79% of American women initiate breastfeeding.

Dr. Jung rails against pumping because pumping time is unpaid. She does not seem to understand that unpaid pumping time is not the real problem; rather, it's that most American mothers do not get paid mater-nity leave as many new mothers do in other countries. Canada does have guaranteed paid maternity leave for up to 18 months (12 months when Dr Jung wrote this article). However, the amount of money mothers receive in Canada is inadequate if you are not already relatively affluent; It may not be enough to cover expenses if their partners are not employed. Some countries, such as the Czech Republic, Slovakia, Hungary, do much better and are less affluent than the USA or Canada.

Dr. Jung doubts studies that show breastfeeding protects against ill-ness, claiming that the studies are methodologically unsound (per her degree in political science). She minimizes the effects of breastfeeding on ear infections, for example. The director of the Agency for Healthcare Research and Quality told her that if six babies exclusively breastfeed for

6 months, only one baby will avoid an ear infection. She exclaims, "That's about 5,400 hours of breastfeeding to prevent one ear infection." She pronounces breastfeeding a waste of time. But is it?

Let's look at this another way. If that 79% of the 3.8 million babies born in the U.S. in 2019 were breastfed, many only did breastfeed for a few days or weeks. Only 25%, or 950,000, were exclusively breastfed to 6 months. [The actual breastfeeding numbers in the U.S. are not quite this good, based on PRAMS data (Ahluwalia, Morrow, & Hsia, 2005).] We really doubt this statistic of 25% *exclusively* breastfed to 6 months but will accept it for the sake of argument.) If that were true, it means that there were 160,000 (!) fewer ear infections in 2019 alone (only 1 in 6 according to the director of the Agency for Healthcare Research and Quality). Clearly, Dr. Jung has never had an ear infection if she can be so relaxed about how much they hurt. Furthermore, many babies are admitted to hospital because they seem worrisomely sick with fever, and it turns out to be an ear infection. Babies with fever younger than 3 months of age are considered high risk for severe illness and septicemia, and thus, they are admitted to the hospital if they have a fever.

As a pediatrician, I (JN) know a lot of exclusively breastfed babies and none of them ever had an ear infection (okay, that's not a study). Here is a secret, and please don't spread it around: when a baby has a fever, the doctor often diagnoses an ear infection. It's a good excuse to prescribe antibiotics and send the parents and baby home. Everyone, including the doctor, but perhaps not the baby, is relieved. This, *perhaps*, can explain why 5 out of 6 exclusively breastfed babies supposedly had ear infections.

Then comes the zinger. Dr. Jung gives scant attention to formula marketing but notes that breastfeeding "is also driven in part by big business — including the companies that manufacture breast pumps, the companies that make nutritional supplements for breastfeeding mothers and babies, and the companies that sell breastfeeding accessories."

I (JN) heard her speak at a Toronto library. She was outraged that pumps and pump rentals cost $4.5 billion and year. This was her *real* pet peeve, though why this should unnerve her so much is beyond me. Apparently, she is *not* outraged by the $45 billion (US) that formula companies sold worldwide that year (2015), risen to $62.5 billion in 2020.

As for nutritional supplements for the baby, they are completely unnecessary; everything that babies need is already in breastmilk. As for "breastfeeding accessories," Dr. Jung means special clothes and pillows. In truth, all you need to breastfeed is a breast and a baby. We find that pillows can cause breastfeeding problems because the baby is often at the wrong height and special clothes usually aren't necessary. These products are not breastfeeding's fault.

She then praises companies like Medela for supporting breastfeeding research, stating that their sponsorship does not deny the results, but they do have a "vested" interest. Not true of legitimate studies! Researchers of *legitimate* studies do not accept sponsorship by companies that have a vested interest in the question. Oddly, she doesn't worry that many studies on "special formulas" are sponsored by vested interests.

## Conclusions

We wanted to open this section by acknowledging that many believe that breastfeeding can potentially cause great harm to infants. Yes, they are vulnerable, especially in the first few days of life, but skilled lactation care and support makes all the difference. The chapters in this section describe what to look for in the early days. Our goal is to help you confidently support mothers and babies in the early days and know how to spot potential problems.

# CHAPTER 6

# Birth Interventions

The medical profession has turned labor and birth into a highly medicalized, unnatural event. It is unusual, in most hospitals, to have a normal, unmedicated birth. True, before there were medical interventions, it was not rare that mothers, babies, or both died in labor. However, even with birth interventions, maternal mortality is actually rising, especially in the U.S., and especially among women of color.

The return of trained midwives who help mothers birth their babies without unnecessary interventions shows that many mothers do not want highly medicalized labors and births. Not surprisingly, birth interventions can interfere with initiating breastfeeding and making breastfeeding work. We would like to briefly describe a few interventions that can make breastfeeding in the hospital more difficult.

## Intravenous Fluids

Hospital births often include an intravenous infusion to maintain the mother's blood pressure in case it drops, or she has significant bleeding. Mothers often receive much more intravenous fluid than is required.

One of our patients, a nurse herself, told the hospital staff nurse *after* her transfer to her room after the baby's birth, that she was receiving too much fluid. The nurse did not listen, so the new mother slowed down the intravenous infusion herself. Later, her nurse returned and upped the intravenous infusion rate while the new mother slept. The mother went into congestive heart failure from fluid overload. Granted, this is a rare situation, but surely less aggressive fluid management is generally possible and desirable.

If mothers receive a lot of intravenous fluids during labor, *so do their babies* since, until the baby is born and the umbilical cord separates or is cut, mother and baby are still one physiologically. This can make the babies weigh more at birth than their true weight; fluid weight that they quickly shed in their urine. This "weight loss" frequently leads to unnecessary supplements. We describe this in more detail in Chapter 7.

## Epidurals

Epidurals can affect babies' ability to breastfeed for several reasons. Epidurals restrict the woman in labor's movement so they cannot easily walk around as many women in labor would like to do. Thus, women in labor are usually lying down or sitting up in bed, which may slow down labor and increase the "need" of other interventions, such as synthetic oxytocin (Pitocin). Epidurals may cause women's blood pressure to drop, which means more IV fluid, and the lower blood pressure may result in less blood getting to babies, which, in turn, may cause distress in the baby. Synthetic oxytocin, another factor resulting in women in labor retaining more fluid, which may then result in breasts becoming swollen with fluid as in the photo below.

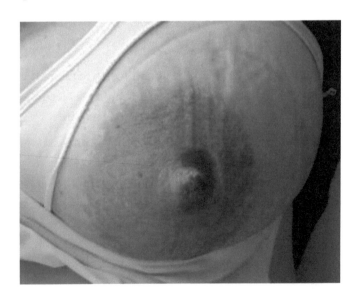

This swelling can make it difficult for babies to latch on well, or not at all. (Note the scab on the mother's nipple from the baby's poor latch.) This swelling of the nipple and areola explains why so many babies have difficulty latching on in the days immediately after birth.

Epidurals can also cause mothers a great deal of pain. Sometimes the needle used to inject anesthetic into the epidural space punctures the membrane that surrounds the spinal cord. This may result in a "spinal" headache, which may be quite severe as fluid leaks out around the lining surrounding the spinal cord. Such pain may keep the new mother from breastfeeding. Spinal headaches can last for several days. Many new mothers are incapacitated by the headache, which is worse if they sit up. Although lying down, side by side with the baby is a good way to breastfeed, no one seems to show new mothers this position in hospital. The mothers' need to lie down flat makes breastfeeding awkward. Doctors may also tell mothers that they cannot have pain medication, *which is not true* (see Chapter 20).

Anesthetists generally insist that the medications they use do not reach the baby. Unfortunately, we now know that epidural medications cross the placenta and negatively affect babies (Beilin et al., 2005; Brimdyr et al., 2015; Moises et al., 2005; Ransjo-Arvidson et al., 2001; Torvaldsen, Roberts, Simpson, Thompson, & Ellwood, 2006; Wiklund, Norman, Uvnas-Moberg, Ransjo-Arvidson, & Andolf, 2009).

My (JN) experience is obviously not a study, but I observed newborn babies in the Transkei (South Africa) when I worked there from 1981 to 1983. Epidural anaesthesia during labor was rare. Even caesarean sections were done with local anesthesia (and *apparently* were quite effective according to the obstetricians, but then, they were not the ones having the caesarean section). Babies were not immediately put skin to skin on the mother, but they were almost always very ready to latch on and breastfeed even though they were washed and wrapped in blankets. Canadian mothers, in contrast, frequently have epidurals and not infrequently, their babies are not ready to latch on. Often, the babies are sleepy, sometimes floppy, and not interested in the breast at all.

### Maternal Fevers

Epidurals can cause fever in mothers (Segal, 2010), which can trigger a chain-reaction of hospital staff response. Mother and baby often are treated with antibiotics, and they are often separated, with the baby going to the neonatal intensive care unit. Unfortunately, antibiotics do not treat viral infections, and separating mothers and babies does not keep babies from getting sick. The mother and baby have been in close contact with their febrile mothers for at least several hours before birth. If fevers do mean an infection, breastfeeding helps to protect the baby.

Pumping is not the same as keeping the mother and baby together and can seriously undermine breastfeeding. Furthermore, previously expressed breastmilk loses some of its anti-microbial elements (such as white cells). Even worse, in many institutions, doctors may not want to use the mother's milk for fear of passing on the possible infection to the baby. The best bet is to keep mothers together, breastfeeding, even if the new mother has fever.

## The Breast Crawl and Skin to Skin

Normal, unmedicated babies are ready at birth to start breastfeeding. Babies put skin to skin on the mother's abdomen after birth exhibit a sequence of behaviors that leads them to crawl up from their mother's abdomen and latch on to the breast. This is similar to the sequence other mammals exhibit (Widstrom et al., 2011). An anecdote: When I did my exam to be registered in Canada as a pediatrician, I mentioned having the new baby on the mother's abdomen so that the baby would crawl to the breast. Both examining pediatricians laughed and said "on the mother's chest, not abdomen. How will the baby crawl from the abdomen?"

Babies can crawl to the breast even a few weeks after birth, if, for some reason, it cannot be done immediately at birth. Skin-to-skin contact is one the triggering mechanisms for the breast crawl and releases oxytocin in both mother and baby. As an aside, skin-to-skin contact is one reason why we recommend using a lactation aid to supplement the baby at the breast, rather than supplement with an open cup, a bottle, finger-feeding, when supplementation is deemed necessary. This way, breastfeeding continues even if babies are not getting enough milk from their mothers.

Watching babies crawl to the breast is magical and much more useful than observing them in the neonatal intensive care unit. After all, a baby with the wherewithal to crawl up his mother's body, find the breast and latch on without help is unlikely to be terribly ill. However, even well babies may not be able to crawl to the breast because epidural drugs keep them from crawling and latching on without help. And some are just not given the time to do it, as it takes an average of almost an hour for the whole process.

## Kangaroo Mother Care (KMC)

Researchers in Colombia first described Kangaroo Mother Care (KMC) in the medical literature in the early 1980s. We are amazed when we find that there are pediatricians and neonatologists who still do not know about the breast crawl, skin-to-skin contact, and Kangaroo Mother Care (KMC). In the original studies, premature babies in Kangaroo Mother Care survived better than those kept in incubators. In fact, they survived better *at home* than babies kept in hospital tended by neonatologists and skilled nursing staff. At first this was put down to the fact that Colombia is a developing economy, but then we started to see the same thing in affluent countries like Sweden, Denmark, and South Africa (Bergman, Linley, & Fawcus, 2004; Nyqvist et al., 2010). Since that time, hundreds of articles have been published from all over the world, showing the benefits to babies' survival, and from our point of view, to breastfeeding as well. A Cochrane Review (Conde-Agudelo & Diaz-Rossello, 2014) found that Kangaroo Mother Care reduced mortality and morbidity in low birthweight infants. Unfortunately, in much of the affluent world, Kangaroo Mother Care is simply not done. Or it may be done in an extremely limited or token amount. In a 20-year longitudinal study, Charpak and colleagues (2017) found that Kangaroo Mother Care had long-lasting effects on babies' social and behavioral development.

The World Health Organization (2003)C produced a guide called *Kangaroo Mother Care: A practical approach*, which you can find by following the link in the reference section.

## Conclusions

Birth interventions can substantially influence breastfeeding, especially intravenous fluids and epidurals. Epidurals can cause pain for mothers and the medications get to babies, making it more difficult for them to latch on. The breast crawl and Kangaroo Mother Care can lower mothers' and babies' stress and can help breastfeeding get on track.

## CHAPTER 7

# Dehydration and Weight Loss after Birth

In hospitals throughout North America (and elsewhere), hospital staff consider newborns who lose 10% or more of their birthweight at risk for dehydration. Hospital staff commonly intervene by giving formula, usually by bottle. In our opinion, this 10% rule, and everything that happens in its wake, is pseudoscience. Unfortunately, practitioners follow along because they are afraid of what will happen if they don't intervene.

The *Washington Post* prides itself on avoiding sensational stories and focusing only on "real" news. Yet, they published this: "She listened to her doctors—and her baby died. Now she's warning others about breast-feeding" (Bever, 2017). This case was undeniably tragic but talk about a sensational and terrifying headline! The mother and baby in this story are victims of horribly inept practice but the author assumed that this baby's death was caused by the mother breastfeeding. In the article the mother is reported to have said,

> It was really hard for me to comprehend that point because I had been breast-feeding him — "What do you mean he was dehy-drated?" Jillian Johnson said she told the doctor in February 2012. "I couldn't wrap my head around it. I was frustrated with myself because, there were these doctors and nurses who kept telling me, 'Just keep feeding him. Just keep him on the breast. You've got a great latch. You're doing fine.'"

The problem was that the baby was not receiving milk, and nobody noticed. They all assumed that if the baby was sucking at the breast, the baby was receiving milk, but obviously, the baby was not receiving much milk at all. Someone who was trained to watch the baby at the breast would have immediately recognized that the baby was not receiving milk, but no one did until it was too late. The article goes on to state: "Then there's the physical pain some women say they endure to breastfeed their babies," and therein lies this case's first flaming clue.

> Johnson, Landon's mother, said that during the three days she was constantly nursing her son, her breasts were sore, and her nipples were raw and bleeding.

When will health professionals ever learn? Breastfeeding *should not hurt!* The mother's bleeding nipples were "shouting out" that something was very wrong. Yet no one came to this mother's aid. If anything, cases like this heighten the urgency of what we have been saying throughout this book and for years in teaching breastfeeding. Breastfeeding "support" is not just "you're doing a great job" pep talks. Health professionals must know how to assess if breastfeeding is going well or not or get someone in who does know how to help the mother and baby. It is not enough for doctors and nurses to say, "the baby is sucking, so he must be getting milk." That is so obviously wrong!

The mother also had sore breasts, which the doctors *thought* meant that she had a lot of milk. Unfortunately, it was another missed sign that something was wrong. *Breasts should not be painful*, not even when the milk "comes in" and the mother's breasts are engorged. Engorged breasts also suggest babies are not drinking well from the breast.

Naturally, the physician/founder of an anti-breastfeeding organization had to comment. She pointed out that the baby lost *almost* 10% of its weight in the first 3 days. We believe that weight alone cannot determine whether babies are drinking well at the breast, especially in the first few days after birth. As always, prevention is the best treatment. Mothers should get good hands-on help as soon as possible after birth. Babies should be *drinking* from the first time they latch on immediately after birth. Watch this video of a 10-hour-old baby who is drinking at the breast after adjustment of the latch and the use of breast compressions.

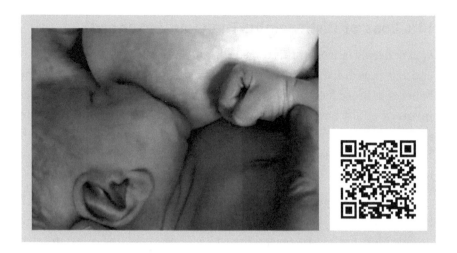

Furthermore, the pediatrician quoted in the article said the following, clearly indicating that breastfeeding usually does not work.

"I'm definitely going to encourage breast-feeding when possible," Bernstein said. (authors' note: we love "when possible"). He further states, "We easily get the majority of our patients breast-feeding, but there is still a significant number of patients who, for a variety of issues, breast-feeding just doesn't work out. As gung-ho as we are about breast-feeding in 2017, I think it has to be done carefully."

This stands as a completely inane remark in response to the tragedy that occurred. And to top things off, he states, "formula is very acceptable source, both alone or to supplement breast milk." What on earth has this to do with anything? In the context of the article, it is, in fact, a strong endorsement for formula-feeding. This statement reminds me of a scene in a Macedonian film called *Before the Rain*. A novice priest is expelled from his community for an unacceptable sin. The head of the community slaps him across the face and then embraces him before sending him away.

The article ends with the mother's chilling and sad statement about her own experience,

"I am not against breast-feeding; I am pro-breastfeeding," she said. "That's the one thing I don't appreciate is everyone saying I need to stop being anti-breastfeeding. I am not. Honestly, if I was anti-breastfeeding, my kid would probably be alive."

## 10% Loss of Birthweight: The Gold Standard?

We are deeply moved by this tragedy. We are also frustrated because it was entirely *preventable*. Unfortunately, tragic cases like these have sown the belief that breastfeeding is *dangerous and risky*. The doctors and nurses involved could have responded by learning something about how to assess the adequacy of breastfeeding and whether things are going well. Instead, they cling to the 10% weight loss as an accurate barometer of infant well-being.

In the last decade or so, the 10% rule has spread like a virus through hospitals in a useless effort to prevent dehydration. Well, it may prevent dehydration, but it also prevents breastfeeding success. The rule states that babies should not lose more than 10% of their birthweight in the first few days. Where this "rule" came from is a mystery. From our perspective, it makes no sense to depend on percentage of weight loss. It is not a good measure of how the breastfeeding is going. Even so, both Baby-Friendly USA and the American Academy of Pediatrics both seem to believe that anything less than 10% means that nothing is amiss. Over 10% is a problem.

### Scale Can Be Unreliable

We have a few serious issues with using 10% as the sole gauge of the adequacy of breastfeeding in the first few days of life. First of all, rules about 10% weight loss assume that scales are accurate or that the person weighing the baby makes no errors in recording the weight. In the "real" world, we should not assume that to be the case. Scales often weigh differently. We have seen significant differences between two different scales (see photos below). One scale is more modern and "accurate looking" than the other, but no two scales should be as different as in the two photos below. The same baby was weighed on two different scales only seconds apart. Clearly one scale is incorrect. In fact, both could be. In the photo on the top, the baby weighs 3.51 kg (7 pounds 11.8 ounces). In the photo on the bottom, the same baby weighs 3.11 kg (6 pounds 13.7 ounces), a difference of 400 grams (or 14 ounces), or a weight loss of more than 11%.

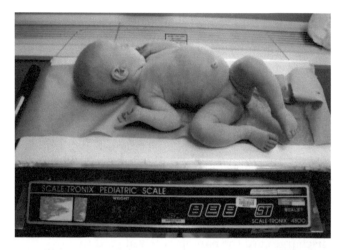

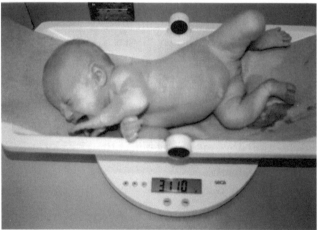

True, it is unusual for two scales to give such disparate results. Incidentally, the one on the top is correct; medical engineers checked it using several different verified weights. We have seen two scales of the same make and model, sitting side by side, that show a difference of 90 grams (3 ounces) weight in the same baby weighed within a minute. When discussing percentage weight loss, 90 grams difference in a 3 kg (6 pounds, almost 9 ounces) baby is a 3% difference that simply depends on the scale.

Even more mistakes can occur when babies are weighed on two different scales. Take, for example, the hospital scale and the one at the doctor's office. If there is a suspicious difference, the results need to be taken with a grain of salt. Yet so many of our patients have been supplemented merely because the baby weighed less on the doctor's scale compared to the hospital scale. Even at the hospital, two scales may produce very different weights.

There's more. People, even highly trained health professionals, occasionally make mistakes. If health professionals are working in pounds and ounces, the calculation of 10% weight loss is not straightforward. Furthermore, sometimes even well-trained physicians or nurses weigh babies and write down the wrong number or make a mistake when they may transfer it into the chart. Here is an example that we documented from the discharge card the parents received (and we saw).

> The baby weighed 2.58 kg (5lb 11oz) at birth and five *hours* later weighed 3.1 kg (6lb 13oz). Clearly there is something that does not make sense here. The pediatrician and nurses undoubtedly agreed that there was an error somewhere, since it would be unusual for a baby weighed again only 5 hours after birth. In fact, what happened was the nurse who admitted the baby to the postpartum ward realized that the baby looked a lot bigger than 2.58 kg and decided to weigh the baby again. (The nurses have a lot of experience, since this hospital has, on average, 100 or more births a week).

What would have happened if the numbers were reversed, and the baby "weighed" 3.1 kg at birth and 2.58 kg the next day? (A decrease of 16.8% in the birthweight). Panic, undoubtedly, amongst the hospital staff. They would have immediately supplemented with formula. This is often the first step on the road that ends breastfeeding. Parents are frightened by, "my baby was dehydrated and could possibly have become quite sick!" In our clinic, we have babies who started formula supplementation on day 2 because of 10% weight loss. Nobody ever seems to ask how a baby can lose so much weight in less than 24 hours. The above situation is not theoretical.

We have other examples from our clinic. There were several instances when weights were obviously incorrect, even when the baby was weighed on the same scale (we have only one). The most egregious example is a baby in 2020 who gained a kilogram (2 lbs 3 oz) in 7 days. Clearly, this cannot be right. We hope you agree. Conversely, we've had a baby who did not gain any weight in 1 week. We asked the mother for details. According to the mother, he was content and happy between feedings, with no real problem. We observed the baby at the breast, and he was drinking well, beautifully, in fact. The next week, we brought the mother and baby back to reassure both the family and us. The baby gained the "requisite" amount of weight in that week. That baby continued to drink well and receive lots of milk. This time, the weight gain verified our observations. Our clinic is usually quite busy, and "busy" can lead to errors.

## Intravenous Fluids Given to Mothers

As we described in the previous chapter, during labor, mothers are frequently given intravenous fluids, which also go to the baby. Thus, babies are frequently born "overhydrated," which may dramatically increase their birthweights. Even if correctly measured at birth, these babies lose weight in the first 24 hours as they urinate this extra fluid (Chantry, Nommsen-Rivers, Peerson, Cohen, & Dewey, 2011).

We used to do this with formula-fed babies back when few babies were breastfed. The rule was that babies should not lose more than 10% of birthweight before starting to gain and should be back to birthweight by 10 days of age. Doctors then applied this rule to breastfed babies and it resulted in many receiving unnecessary supplements. Why did they apply it to breastfeeding babies? Probably because it was easier to look at numbers rather than attempt to evaluate a baby at the breast.

Ten percent has also become a slippery slope. Instead of the 10% weight loss being a problem, it becomes, "Well, 9% is almost 10%, so we should supplement the baby, and 8% is almost 9% etc., etc."). We've even seen some hospitals recommend supplement following a 5% weight loss in the first 24 hours. The message? Start supplements on day 1. That is absurd, but it is exactly what it is happening. We believe that knowing how to know a baby is *drinking at the breast* is an important skill, important not only for the health professional, but also for the mother, but it is clearly not taught, because who is going to teach it? It is rare, and we choose that word carefully, that a mother referred to our clinic has even an inkling of how to know a baby is drinking at the breast.

### More Tyranny of 10% Weight Loss

Relying solely on weight as an indicator to intake also scares parents. We received this email from a mother of a 17-week-old baby. He was mostly bottle-feeding. He might take the breast a little, only occasionally, but the baby was getting only breastmilk and gaining.

> Think I got off to a bad start...the nurse told me my baby was losing too much weight (not even 10 percent of her birthweight in hindsight) and told me to get pumping. *"I have been worried ever since"* (our italics)

This is what we are doing to mothers with our emphasis on numbers and weights, trusting only the scale, instead of helping the mother achieve a good latch and watching the baby at the breast. This mother has been "worried ever since," and she now may consider her baby a "vulnerable child," which can lead to developmental symptoms.

## Observing Babies at the Breast: The Better Metric

We contend that the scale is a poor indicator of how well the baby is breastfeeding. Observing the baby at the breast is far more important than weighing babies. At the very least, the weights need to be confirmed by history and, most importantly, *observation*. The scale should agree with the history and observation.

The real problem is that many hospital staff, physicians, pediatricians, midwives, postpartum nurses do not know what to look for. Super Clue #1: if the mother has sore nipples, then the baby is not latched on well. Just because painful breastfeeding in the first days is common does not mean that it is normal or acceptable, "everyone has it"; it is not, *and the mother and baby require good help, then and there.*

Perhaps worse when the baby is not latching on well, the baby does not get milk well, falls asleep at the breast, and has to be vigorously stimulated to wake up. More likely, he will have a bottle of formula forced into his mouth. Yes, that will wake him up, but why was the problem not noted *before* the baby became difficult to wake up? Unfortunately, many babies get supplemented when they are actually doing well breastfeeding, based only on change in weight. Conversely, babies who may need help don't receive it because the scale says the weight gain is good.

## When Supplementation Is Necessary

In our experience, "emergency" formula supplementation would not occur if hospital staff knew how to assess whether babies are drinking well at the breast, or not, or something in between. Unfortunately, it seems that very few postpartum staff are well trained in evaluating the adequacy of breastfeeding. Even when they are, they may be overruled by protocols written by pediatricians and neonatologists who have never themselves watched a baby at the breast with the idea of evaluating how well the baby is drinking.

If supplementation is needed, we suggest using the mother's own milk as a first choice, then banked or donated breastmilk or physiological water (water with electrolytes and glucose). All these choices are better than formula. If the concern is dehydration, then why not physiological water? Unfortunately, giving formula sends parents a strong message: *this is the good stuff.* Your baby needs it. It saved your baby from mortal danger. Agreed, formula may be necessary in some situations, but we suggest using it only after other approaches have been tried. Ordinary formula has *very little* in common with more mature breastmilk, never mind with colostrum. In addition, the use of bottles may cause the baby to refuse to latch on.

### Alternatives to Bottle-Feeding

Bottles are another problem. We generally suggest avoiding bottles, especially in the first few days, because they can influence how the baby latches on to the breast and possibly cause the baby to prefer the bottle and even refuse to take the breast completely. Below, we list alternative ways of feeding babies who need supplementation.

### Lactation Aid at the breast

In a few hospitals, mothers are offered a lactation aid to supplement. If the staff do not know how to show mothers the proper use of the lactation aid, mothers are frustrated by the time they see us. When *we* see mothers, their first reaction is, "Don't even talk about it. It does not work. And I am completely stressed out about using it." Actually, used correctly, it works very well, but it may take some practice. The photo below shows a baby being supplemented at the breast with a lactation aid (with formula).

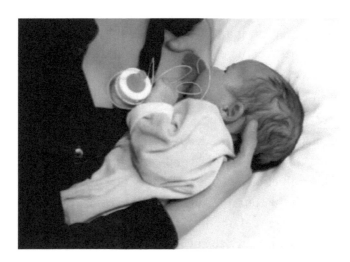

### Cup Feeding

Cup feeding does not help improve latch, but it does not interfere with the latch as much as bottles do. Cup feeding keeps the baby well hydrated until the mother can get good help with latching on the baby. A recent review indicated that babies fed by cup were slightly more likely to breastfeed exclusively compared to those fed with bottles (McKinney et al., 2016). Premature babies who were cup fed had higher oxygen saturations and few problems with desaturation.

### Finger Feeding

Midwives in our area sometimes favor finger feeding, but we have reservations. If the baby will latch on to the breast and needs supplementation, then a lactation aid at the breast would be the best approach. The mother's own breastmilk is by far the first choice of supplement, or, if necessary, banked breastmilk or donated breastmilk. If none of these is available, then physiological water (meaning water with some electrolytes and glucose) would be superior to formula. After all, we are concerned about *dehydration*, not necessarily making sure the baby gets enough "food." Most babies will be fine for several days as long as they remain well hydrated while we help the baby to latch on well. In fact, many NICUs give dehydrated babies intravenous physiologic water. That the first choice of supplement in the first few days is formula speaks volumes on the breastfeeding support most mothers and babies receive in the immediate postpartum period.

While we do not like finger feeding as a primary feeding mechanism, it works well to help a baby who is not latching on to latch on.

## Conclusion

Dehydration is an important symptom to monitor, but weight loss is not the best way to monitor it. Weight loss is highly susceptible to human error in weighing and is not a substitute for a complete history and observing the baby at the breast, especially observing the baby at the breast. It's critical that mothers, and all healthcare professionals they encounter, know how to assess whether babies are drinking well at the breast.

# CHAPTER 8

# Hypoglycemia

Persistent hypoglycemia (low blood glucose) in newborns (or anyone for that matter) is serious and can cause irreversible brain damage. All health professionals who work with infants know this. It most commonly occurs in the first 24 hours. Because of these risks, hospitals take what we would call an unreasoned approach to preventing and treating it. But what exactly is hypoglycemia?

Surprisingly, there is no universally accepted definition of hypoglycemia in newborns (Cornblath et al., 2000). Numbers for the lower level of glucose range from 2.5 mmol/L (45 mg%) to 3.0 mmol/L (54 mg%) in various postpartum care units in Toronto hospitals. Some U.S. hospitals recommend an even higher minimum glucose (probably to be "safe" and perhaps, to avoid getting sued). Furthermore, there is no *accurate* bedside method of measuring plasma glucose. Bedside methods measure *blood* glucose, which underestimates the more accurate *plasma* glucose. In addition, asymptomatic hypoglycemia does not appear to damage full-term healthy newborns (Cornblath et al., 2000). Therefore, there is no reason for universal screening of normal newborns (Hoseth, Joergensen, Ebbesen, & Moeller, 2000).

## Maternal Diabetes as a Risk Factor

Newborns at the highest risk for low blood glucose are those whose mothers have diabetes (either type). Diabetes may cause high blood glucose levels during pregnancy, resulting in high blood glucose for the fetus. Because mothers may have high blood glucose levels during pregnancy, babies produce insulin, something the mother, especially the mother with type 1 diabetes, cannot do. Insulin is a hormone that, in addition to lowering the glucose, also causes more tissue and fat to be deposited in the baby's body.

Once these babies are born, the babies' pancreas continues to produce *increased* insulin levels for about 24 hours, even though they are no longer receiving high levels of glucose from the mother. Thus, there is a risk that babies' blood glucose will decrease to *lower than normal* levels. These levels might be so low as to cause brain damage especially if the low blood sugar is *persistent and not corrected.*

## Large (or Small) for Gestational Age

Babies whose mothers have diabetes may be born large for gestational age (LGA). LGA usually defined as weighing more than 90% of babies at birth. On the other hand, if the pregnant woman's diabetes is persistently and drastically out of control, the baby may be smaller than expected at birth, although this scenario is unlikely if she is receiving good prenatal care.

Unfortunately, *any* baby who is born larger than expected is often considered to be at risk for low blood glucose, even if the mother did not have diabetes during the pregnancy. Somebody, somebody normal, must be over the 90th percentile, by definition. However, if mothers did not have gestational diabetes, their larger babies are *not* at risk for low blood glucose simply because they are bigger than most other babies at birth. In fact, these babies are quite capable of maintaining their blood glucose, by mobilizing glycogen, which is abundantly stored in their livers. Glycogen is broken down into its component molecule (glucose) and the baby's blood glucose is maintained. An exception is Beckwith-Wiedemann syndrome, where the baby is born quite large but has other features (large tongue, for example) to tip off the pediatrician that this is not just any large for gestational age baby. These babies have persistent low blood sugar that is often difficult to treat.

There are other situations when the baby *may* be at risk for low blood glucose, including, prematurity and being small for gestational age. Whatever the cause, breastfeeding should be an integral part of the approach to treatment. Mothers can also express milk prenatally if there is concern that the baby might be hypoglycemic soon after birth.

## Blood Glucose Normally Drops

Lactation consultants often are intimidated into going along with aggressive measures to treat low blood glucose because of its potential seriousness. It may help to know that something that many physicians, even pediatricians, do not seem to know. In the first 2 or so hours after birth, blood sugar *normally* drops, sometimes to levels that would be considered low blood glucose or hypoglycemia if this normal variation is not taken into consideration. Indeed, we may have been needlessly treating babies for low blood sugar for the past 50 years, as these Dutch researchers reported in the *New England Journal of Medicine* (van Kempen et al., 2020).

> In this randomized trial involving otherwise healthy newborns, born at 35 weeks or more of gestation and at a birthweight of 2000 g or more, who had asymptomatic moderate hypoglycemia, a management strategy of starting treatment at a glucose concentration threshold of 36 mg per deciliter (2.0 mmol/l) proved noninferior to a strategy that used a threshold of 47 mg per deciliter (2.7 mmol/l) with regard to the infants' psychomotor development at 18 months (p. 543).

There is a good reason for babies' normal drop in blood glucose. Low blood sugar signals adults, and presumably infants, that it is time to eat and likely encourages the first breastfeed in newborns.

However, if someone does not know this and if blood glucose is measured immediately after birth, the normal drop can look like a problem even though it is not harmful. The normal drop is *not* sustained, and will go back up to the normal range *even if the baby is not fed*. Consider this statement by Cornblath and colleagues (2000).

> In the majority of healthy neonates, the *frequently observed low blood glucose concentrations are not related to any significant problem* and merely reflect normal processes of metabolic adaptation to extrauterine life… During the first 2 hours of postnatal life, there is a decline in plasma glucose levels followed by a rise, reaching a steady state glucose concentration by 2 to 3 hours after birth (emphasis added, p. 1141).

## Nature Provides a Backup Plan: Ketone Bodies

Breastfeeding and good intake of breastmilk (watch baby at the breast) is particularly relevant because breastmilk maintains the glucose and increases ketone bodies in the baby's blood. (Cornblath et al., 2000). Ketone bodies protect the brain against the negative effects of low blood glucose. In other words, breastfed babies have a higher concentration of ketone bodies, which also nourish the brain and prevent brain damage. It's not just about glucose!

## No Need to Separate Mothers at Risk for Low Blood Glucose

Unfortunately, too often, treating possible low blood glucose results in mothers and babies being separated and the baby being transferred to the neonatal intensive care unit. In most cases, this is not necessary. Indeed, it may add to the problem. For example, Chertok and colleagues (2009) found that infants who breastfed in the delivery room had a significantly lower rate of borderline hypoglycemia than those who were not breastfed in the early postpartum period. Stage et al. (2010) found that even when mothers had type 1 diabetes, newborns who roomed in had reduced morbidity compared to those who had been separated from their mothers. Skin-to-skin contact with the mother immediately after birth encourages latching on. It also helps stabilize blood sugar because it lowers stress.

Of course, if for some reason, the baby's blood glucose is difficult to maintain with breastfeeding and skin to skin alone, then doctors can prescribe an intravenous infusion of glucose, with care not to raise the glucose too abnormally high levels.

On the other hand, glucose gel, *with continued breastfeeding*, can also be used. It has been used for some years in the Great Britain. Better glucose gel than formula, in our opinion. This review from the Canadian Agency for Drugs and Technology in Health (Canadian Agency for Drugs and Technology in Health, Palylyk-Colwell, & Campbell, 2018). supports its use. One of the key points is that oral glucose gel prevents separation of the mothers and babies and allows early initiation of breastfeeding.

## Prenatal Expression of Colostrum

Prenatal expression of colostrum is one way to make sure the baby receives breastmilk immediately after birth. Prenatal expression could even be considered *routine* for all pregnant women. There is milk in the first few days, but if the mother does not get good help in the hospital, her baby might not receive it. We realize that prenatal milk expression diminishes the natural way of breastfeeding, but for now it may be the best way until all healthcare professionals learn what they need to know about breast-feeding (one can dream).

We recommend starting expression at about 35 weeks gestation. Hand expression is usually easiest and often works better than a pump. The photo on the left, below, shows the results of 5 minutes of expression by a mother before the birth of her baby. The second photo shows the total prenatal expression by a mother.

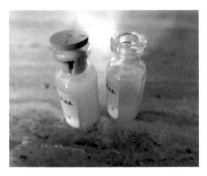 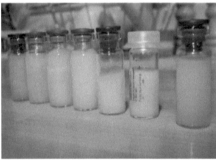

A qualitative study of Australian women (Brisbane & Giglia, 2015) found that most pregnant women and new mothers found prenatal expression to increase,

> … the security that came from having a supply of colostrum that was stored was reassuring for those women who achieved this and may help to alleviate maternal stress over breast milk supply in the immediate postpartum period.

Some criticize prenatal expression because they think that the baby will get less from the breast after birth. We are surprised by this criticism since the breast continually makes milk. In hospitals, babies with possible low blood glucose are "fed" with formula, glucose gel, or intravenous glucose, and not even offered the breast. In addition, mothers and babies might be separated, making it even more difficult for breastfeeding to get off to a good start. Prenatal expression may forestall those events.

## Conclusion

Hypoglycemia is another possible issue that needs to be assessed. Some babies are at higher risk, but hypoglycemia is often over diagnosed, and babies are unnecessarily supplemented with formula. Prevention is key. Babies who are drinking well at the breast are unlikely to have hypoglycemia. Mothers can also ward off possible supplementation with prenatal expression of colostrum that they can bring to the hospital.

## CHAPTER 9

# High Bilirubin and Jaundice

In the immediate postpartum period, typically around Day 3, a significant percentage of newborns show obvious yellowing of the skin that is caused by bilirubin, a compound that originates from the breakdown of old red blood cells. Yellowing of the skin may be more difficult to notice in dark-skinned babies. Historically, high bilirubin has been important to monitor because babies with severe hyperbilirubinemia sometimes had another condition called hemolysis, which led to brain damage and severe chronic illness. In extreme cases, some babies even died.

When the babies who died were autopsied, the medical examiners found yellow staining of the basal ganglia of their brains. Bilirubin was blamed for the brain damage as it is not supposed to be in the brain. But bilirubin may have been, essentially, an innocent bystander. Hemolysis is the actual culprit. Hemolysis, and its attendant abnormalities broke down the blood-brain barrier and allowed bilirubin to enter the brain. Hypoxia, hypoglycemia, acidosis, and the other metabolic abnormalities damaged babies' brains.

## Hemolysis

Hemolysis is a rapid breakdown of the red cells. Red blood cells have a limited life span. In adults, their lifespan is about 120 days, but in the newborn, it's 60 to 90 days. Babies normally have more red cells breaking down at any time, relatively speaking, compared to adults. A more rapid breakdown of the cells, hemolysis, can be caused by several abnormal situations, such as incompatibility of blood types between the mother and baby. ABO incompatibility is the most common type these days, but Rh incompatibility used to be the most common and more severe. Fortunately, it has almost been eliminated by prenatal injections of Rh immune globulin. A condition called G6PD deficiency can also cause hemolysis and extremely high bilirubin levels. G6PD deficiency is most common in babies of Mediterranean and East Asian origin.

If the baby is breastfeeding well, but the bilirubin is rising quickly, hemolysis is likely the cause. Babies with severe hemolysis have more than jaundice and high bilirubin levels. They may also have severe anemia (the only baby I ever saw with Rh incompatibility was admitted to hospital with a hemoglobin of 2 g%, the normal in a newborn being greater than 14 g%). Severe anemia can lead to congestive heart failure. Furthermore, hypoglycemia may occur with Rh incompatibility (due to stress?). Severe anemia may cause acidosis due to poor oxygenation of the baby's tissues.

Sepsis also can cause hemolysis, but babies with sepsis are unlikely to breastfeed well because they are generally very ill. A rise in bilirubin can also occur with a less serious infection, say a urinary tract infection. If infection is causing hemolysis, treating the infection while continuing breastfeeding is indicated. With severe hemolysis, babies may need an exchange transfusion, taking out the baby's blood and replacing it with a compatible blood transfusion.

Both galactosemia and acute viral hepatitis increase the *direct-reacting* bilirubin, and the situation is completely different from the situation of acute hemolysis, which causes indirect hyperbilirubinemia. Most jurisdictions automatically screen for galactosemia at birth and viral hepatitis is very unlikely in newborn babies.

## Monitoring Bilirubin

Considering the possible seriousness of high bilirubin, we might conclude that high bilirubin is always bad, right? The answer is not so straightforward. We used to think that a rise in bilirubin in the first few days was okay and normal if it was not *too* high. Bilirubin levels typically peak around Day 3. We expect a decrease in formula-fed babies because we know they get a lot of milk. In the usual situation, bilirubin decreases after Day 3 and becomes unnoticeable after Days 5 to 7. Of course, formula-fed babies can also have a rapid rise in the bilirubin if they have hemolysis due to an infection or metabolic abnormality, so that is also a cause for concern.

## Does Breastfeeding Cause High Bilirubin?

Some say that bilirubin rises because breastmilk causes it to. Not true. Bilirubin levels of exclusively breastfed babies follow the same trajectory as formula-fed infants *if the breastfed baby takes in adequate amounts of breastmilk.* A rise in bilirubin warns us that the baby may not be breastfeeding well. Insufficient intake, not breastmilk, is the problem. Hospital staff need to help the baby do two things well: latch on and get milk from the breast.

The worst-case scenario is when babies breastfeed so poorly that they become very sleepy. As a result, they breastfeed even less. If the situation continues, the baby does not take the breast at all and seems uninterested in feeding. Many health professionals believe, wrongly, that bilirubin makes babies sleepy. Rather, we believe that lack of breastmilk that makes them sleepy. Case after case has occurred with the baby suffering brain damage due to severe dehydration. Bilirubin and breastmilk are blamed—not the poor breastfeeding and poor intake of breastmilk, with the resulting dehydration and its accompanying abnormalities of acid/base balance. All of these problems could have been avoided with good help with breastfeeding from Day 1.

## Frequency of Bowel Movements

If baby's bowel movements are infrequent, more bilirubin is reabsorbed from the baby's intestinal tract, increasing the levels of serum bilirubin. The most common cause of infrequent bowel movements in newborns is decreased intake of breastmilk. Other causes of increased enterohepatic circulation of bilirubin include congenital hypothyroidism, which causes infrequent bowel movements, or bowel obstruction.

If a 3- or 4-day-old baby has a higher-than-average bilirubin, *it is vital to make sure the baby is breastfeeding well.* If the baby is breastfeeding well, then there is likely no issue if there is no hemolysis or infection. If breastfeeding does not improve, supplement with the mother's breastmilk, banked or donated breastmilk, or physiological water (orally or by intravenous). Formula is an option but should be the *last* choice. Colostrum expressed prenatally is a good supplement that can treat jaundice as well as low blood sugar. If increasing the intake of milk by the baby does not fix the problem, investigate other possible causes, such as infection or a metabolic abnormality.

## "Breastmilk Jaundice"

Breastmilk jaundice is a whole different issue from early-onset jaundice and there is no real relationship between this inappropriate term (breastmilk jaundice) and the early onset jaundice discussed in the previous section. True, early onset jaundice may affect breastfeeding babies in the first few days just as it does artificially fed babies. Exclusively breastfeeding babies 4 to 6 weeks old will often be visibly jaundiced, but there is a huge difference between the two situations. Some babies had early onset *normal* jaundice. They may continue to have obvious jaundice, sometimes for 3 or more months, though it generally diminishes as the weeks go by.

So-called breastmilk jaundice is *not a problem* if the baby is latched on and *drinking well* from the breast, gaining weight well, and there are no signs of liver problems (which causes *conjugated* hyperbilirubinemia, a different sort of jaundice). In this case, "breastmilk jaundice" is *good, not bad* because bilirubin acts as an antioxidant, which decreases babies' risk, amongst other things, of cellular damage and infection, including Group B strep (Hansen et al., 2018; Sedlak & Snyder, 2004).

We follow with two examples of healthy babies with jaundice. The baby in the first photo was born slightly prematurely at 36 weeks gestation. In the photo, he is 6 weeks old. He was born at 2.87 kg (6lb 5oz), and at 6 weeks (on our scale) was 4.57 kg (10lb 1oz). He is exclusively breastfeeding, gaining weight well, and never received anything but breastmilk.

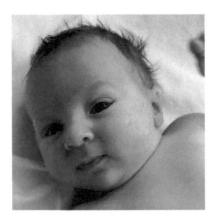

Even more important than good weight gain was the fact that he was drinking very well at the breast, with lots of long pauses in the chin. He fed on both breasts and came off satisfied. The way the baby drinks confirms the weight gain. Without observing a baby at the breast, one cannot tell if the baby is really doing well with breastfeeding.

The baby in the next photo was also breastfeeding exclusively and gaining weight well, but most importantly was drinking very well when we observed him at our clinic. As can be seen in the photo, the baby is jaundiced, but he is also quite chubby.

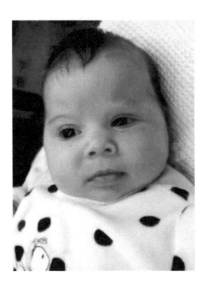

Unfortunately, neither the family doctor, nor her family wanted this mother to continue breastfeeding. She did not follow-up for her next appointment, so we do not know what happened, but we suspect that she did stop breastfeeding. That would be a real shame. Unfortunately, it is not rare that mothers are told to interrupt breastfeeding for "breastmilk jaundice." Typical advice is to interrupt breastfeeding for 2 or 3 days, but some mothers have been told to stop altogether. There is no reason to interrupt breastfeeding at all!

## Biliary Atresia: Important to Rule Out

When a baby is obviously jaundiced at 2 or 4 weeks of life, it is necessary to rule out biliary atresia. Biliary atresia is uncommon (it occurs in about 1 in 10,000 births in the U.S.), but early diagnosis is important; it can be successfully treated if diagnosed early. Biliary atresia causes jaundice in the baby because the duct that connects the liver to the intestinal tract is blocked. Thus, instead of the bile flowing as it normally does into the intestines, the bile (bilirubin) regurgitates back into the blood from the liver. Some is excreted into the urine, which turns it brownish. It also results in lighter bowel movements, although this can be difficult to notice because bowel movements of exclusively breastfed babies are already lighter than those of older children eating a variety of foods.

On physical examination, a baby with biliary atresia will usually have an enlarged, firm liver and possibly an enlarged spleen. Furthermore, testing the baby's urine with a dipstick made for this purpose will usually be positive for bilirubin. The test should not be positive if the baby's jaundice is due to "breastmilk jaundice." If there is any question, the baby's level of serum bilirubin should be tested, measuring not only the usual "indirect reacting" bilirubin seen in breastmilk jaundice, but also the "direct reacting" bilirubin seen in biliary atresia.

We learned one tragic story of biliary atresia. The baby was given formula by bottle in hospital for jaundice. As a result, the baby would not latch on. However, with help from a good lactation consultant, the baby did latch on, and the mother was able to breastfeed exclusively.

At about 3 weeks of age, a doctor saw the baby and told the mother to stop breastfeeding because of breastmilk jaundice. The mother was not happy with this advice and the jaundice continued. The lactation consultant was now alarmed by the brownish urine and recommended continued breastfeeding, but referred the mother and baby to another doctor, who diagnosed biliary atresia. The baby was awaiting liver transplantation but, tragically, died before the planned surgery.

## Gilbert's Syndrome

The idea that bilirubin can be good for a baby (or an adult for that matter) never seems to impose on the thinking of most health professionals. There is a fascinating association of higher-than-average levels of bilirubin in an inherited condition called Gilbert's syndrome and a lower incidence of atherosclerosis (Kundar, Singh, & Bulmer, 2015). Atherosclerosis is now believed to be an inflammatory disease (Fava & Montagnana, 2018). One physician I (JN) trained with in 1970 had Gilbert's syndrome and he lorded it over us because he kept insisting his risk of myocardial infarction was much lower than ours. He always looked as if he had a nice tan year-round.

In fact, people with Gilbert's syndrome are, apparently, otherwise normal in every other way, meaning, no more or less prone to the diseases and health problems of modern life. The jaundice is not always noticeable in such people, but with infection or stress, the bilirubin may rise. Interesting? Maybe. It suggests that in certain situations, bilirubin is a good thing, rising to protect the individual when she or he has an infection of some sort.

## What Is the Bottom Line?

*Neither breastfeeding nor breastmilk causes higher than average bilirubin levels in the first few days after birth.* In fact, the most common reason for higher-than-average bilirubin in the first few days is the baby not breastfeeding well and thus not getting enough breastmilk. So, the first steps are to watch the baby at the breast, to decide if the baby is latched on well and drinking well at the breast. Someone who knows how to evaluate the adequacy of breastfeeding should observe any baby at the breast daily starting on Day 1. Correcting the latch and making sure the baby is drinking at the breast are both very important and will prevent higher levels of bilirubin, and difficulties with breastfeeding in general.

# LATCHING ON AND DRINKING WELL

# CHAPTER 10

# Latch and Drinking at the Breast

It is very frustrating for mothers, families, babies, and us when many health professionals wait weeks before referring mothers and babies to our clinic. In far too many cases, the health professional refuses and simply states that, "formula is just fine." Some mothers can figure things out without expert, experienced help; the majority do not. When a baby cannot (or won't) latch on, and the mother is pumping and feeding her milk in a bottle, it takes skill and lots of experience to turn the situation around. The mother and baby need to be seen within 1 to 2 weeks after the birth. Even 2 weeks is bordering on too long.

It is not difficult to diagnose babies who do not latch on, so we do not understand why some practitioners take up to *3 months* or *even longer*, before sending such mothers and babies to us. What is the point of waiting? Maybe it's because babies are being fed, even if it's in a bottle, so all is well? Unfortunately, most mothers cannot sustain an exclusive pumping regimen for long. Some do, of course, but it's often very difficult for many. There has to be a better way.

While in training, physicians and nurses learn to measure blood pressure and to listen to the heart. They may learn to do a lumbar puncture for diagnosis and to guide treatment. Yet, most health professionals, including many lactation consultants, do not know how to recognize a good latch, even though it's easier to learn than a lot of other things in medicine. In this chapter, we will show you what you need to know.

## Sore Nipples Are *Not* a Normal Part of Breastfeeding

Many health professionals believe that it is normal for breastfeeding mothers to have sore nipples and breasts. It is what mothers "sign up for" when they decide to breastfeed. We strongly disagree! Breastfeeding should not hurt. Sore nipples are common (i.e., a lot of women experience them), but should not be accepted as normal. Nipple pain tells you that something is wrong. Almost certainly the problem relates to how the baby latches on.

If mothers have sore nipples, treatment should be initiated right away by improving the latch and releasing a tongue-tie (if there is one, though in our area, even the tightest of tongue-ties are diagnosed as "mild, unlikely to cause problems"). Sore nipples are much easier to treat when babies are a few days old rather than later and can almost always be successfully treated at this time. This is true in general: the sooner a breastfeeding problem is addressed, the easier it is to overcome.

We cannot imagine the mother's distress when she comes to our clinic and has had sore nipples for 6 weeks or longer. Three months is not rare. On March 22, 2022, we saw a 6-month-old baby whose mother has had sore nipples since the birth of the baby. Our clinic is busy so sometimes mothers must wait for an appointment, but usually not longer than a week. Yes, a week of sore nipples is difficult to sustain for the mother when she has had nipple pain for 3 weeks already, but if the mother continues to have nipple pain on leaving the hospital even if the pain is lessening, she should be referred then and there. Better yet, refer her while she still in the hospital. Sore nipples are bad enough, but a less than adequate latch and sore nipples can lead to blocked ducts, mastitis, and even breast abscess.

Maybe it's because almost everyone believes that breastfeeding is supposed to hurt. Health professionals often dismiss mother's pain and say, "it will get better in a couple of weeks." With all due respect, that's easy for them to say since they are not the ones living the pain. It's true that sore nipples often *do* improve when the mother's milk flow increases, but that may take 3 weeks or even longer. Why should mothers suffer for weeks when effective treatment is available?

Sore nipples can be agonizingly painful. See photo below on the left. The baby is only a day or two old (mother is still in hospital clothing). The mother received *immediate* help for her sore nipples, by getting help to latch the baby on in the best way possible. Her pain was resolved immediately. The mother and baby breastfed for about 3 years with no further problems. The second photo shows the baby latched on with a good, *asymmetric* latch. The third photo shows the baby breastfeeding at 14 months.

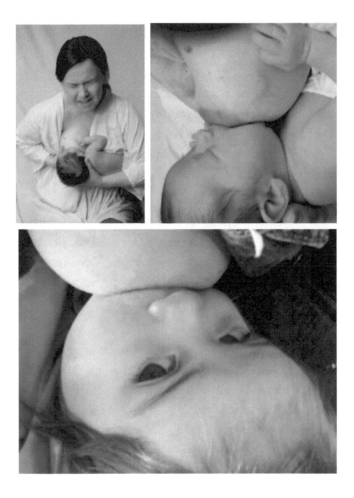

Why does more rapid, more sustained milk flow decrease nipple soreness in many mothers? More rapid, more sustained milk flow improves the baby's latch and a baby latched on better causes less pain.

# What to Do for Sore Nipples

Fortunately, sore nipples are usually easy to address, especially when addressed within a day or two after birth. But even later. Here is what you should try first.

### Improve the Baby's Latch

Make sure babies are latched on well, with an asymmetric latch. Their lower gums should cover more their mothers' areola than their upper gums.

### Improve the Flow

More flow, *faster* flow, results from babies latching on with more breast in their mouths. When babies get a good flow of milk, their latch improves as mentioned above. If flow is slow, babies tend to slip down on the breast, latching on only on the nipple, which causes mothers pain.

### Release Tongue-Ties

Tongue-tie, if present, should be released as soon as possible after the birth of the baby. We believe that tight tongue-ties should be released prophylactically on Day 1, even when mothers have no pain. Releasing the tongue-tie also helps babies get more milk in the first few days.

### Candida Infection?

Candida ("yeast," or "thrush") is not a usual cause of nipple pain. At least, it is not a primary cause. Candida does not grow on normal, undamaged skin, but can cause problems in the folds of skin when moisture accumulates. Candida does not cause nipple pain unless skin is already damaged. A baby's poor latch damages the skin and thus the way the baby latches on is the first thing that needs to be addressed.

## All-Purpose Nipple Ointment (APNO)

APNO is an ointment that I (JN) developed as a temporary measure to decrease nipple pain, but it is not a substitute for good "hands on help." (Not everyone likes the term "hands on help," but it is a convenient term.) As the name of the ointment implies, it is *all purpose*. It helps most mothers, whatever the cause of soreness. But it is *not* a definite treatment. It is a temporary treatment until the baby's latch can be adjusted, including by releasing a tongue-tie. APNO is made up by the pharmacist and contains:

1. Mupirocin ointment 2%: 15 grams. This antibiotic kills *Staphylococcus aureus as well as other bacteria.*

2. Betamethasone ointment 0.1%: 15 grams. This corticosteroid decreases inflammation. A corticosteroid ointment alone was used for years for the treatment of sore nipples, but with only variable success.

3. Miconazole powder 2%. This antifungal agent treats Candida. If powdered miconazole is not available, as it is not in many countries, such as Great Britain, it can be left out if the other ingredients are available.

    →total is 30 grams +/-

I (JN) always write "No Substitutions" at the bottom of the prescription to avoid inappropriate pharmacist substitutions.

### APNO Is a Stop-Gap Measure Only

Hospital pharmacists in our area tell mothers to not use APNO for more than 2 weeks. Their concern is "thinning of the skin," a well-known side effect of topical corticosteroids. However, we have *never* seen this in any of our patients, and it is a shame to stop the ointment just as things are improving. If mothers are not able to get help quickly with the latch or a tongue-tie release, they may need to keep using it until they can get help.

## How to Evaluate Latch

Here is how to evaluate latch. To begin with, let us we consider the same baby latched on well and less well.

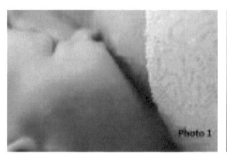 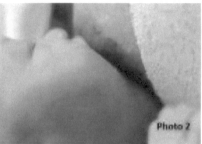

Photo 1 (on the left) shows the baby latched on in a traditional, *symmetric* latch, which can work well enough, especially if the mother produces a lot of milk, and the mother is not in pain. Photo 2 (on the right) shows an *asymmetric latch,* which is much better. There is more space between the baby's nose and the breast and the baby's head is more tilted back. The baby's lower lip covers more of the areola than his upper lip, and the nipple is pointing more towards the roof of the baby's mouth. The asymmetric latch works better because there is more breast over the baby's *lower* gums; it is the lower part of the mouth (the mandible) that moves and stimulates the release of milk.

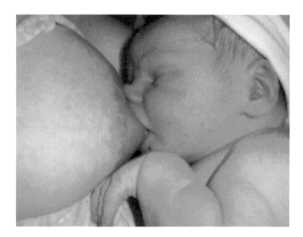

The above photo shows a truly poor latch. The baby has an asymmetric latch, true enough, but it is the opposite of a *good* asymmetric latch. The baby covers more of the areola with his *upper gum* than the *lower gum*. The baby's lower gums are over the nipple, which will cause the mother pain, and cannot stimulate the breast to release milk, because the lower gums are too far away from the breast tissue. On the other hand, the baby's upper jaw *does not move* and thus cannot stimulate release of milk. The mother and baby in this photo are on the way to serious problems: sore nipples and not enough milk.

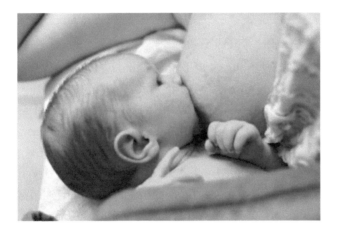

This baby's latch is also not a good one but not as wildly poor as the previous baby. The baby covers more of the areola with his maxilla, *which does not move,* than with the mandible which *does* move. This baby will have difficulty stimulating the breast so that, as a result, the milk is less likely to flow well. However, if the mother produces a lot of milk, the breastfeeding *may* go well enough, though milk production and flow may decrease with time.

## How to Know If the Baby Is Drinking at the Breast

The baby's latch is the first part of the equation. The second is drinking well at the breast. Too many believe that if babies are latched on and making sucking movements, they must be drinking milk. This is not necessarily true. A baby may latch on, drink for a bit, and then "nibble" for the rest of the time. If the baby does not gain weight, healthcare professionals will usually tell mothers to supplement, and usually with a bottle which will not improve the baby's latch at all. In fact, it may worsen how the baby latches on.

Unfortunately, some doctors believe low weight gain is because women's milk is "too weak." The real problem is that most doctors, *especially* pediatricians, do not watch the baby at the breast. Usually, even if they do watch the baby on the breast, they don't know what to watch for. That is why *mothers, and their partners* need to know how to know the baby is drinking at the breast.

## When Babies Are Drinking Well

The 3-week-old baby in the video below, had never latched on to the breast until this visit to our clinic. The video shows a baby drinking well at the breast, clearly getting lots of milk. The baby's chin pauses as he opens his mouth to the widest point. This pause, each pause, indicates that the baby is receiving a goodly amount of milk. The *longer* the pause, the *more milk* the baby received. If babies drink like this for several minutes (no numbers please), and come off the breast content, they drank a lot of milk. Mother should offer the other breast, but if the baby does not want the second breast, the baby is probably full.

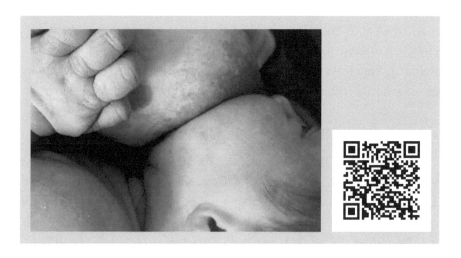

We emphasize that babies should always be offered the second side. If babies are no longer *drinking* on the first side, there is no reason to keep them there nibbling for long periods of time, though on occasion, the mother may have another milk-ejection reflex. Many mothers are being told that the baby should stay on the first side for long periods of time so that the baby receives the "high-fat hind milk." Here is a secret: if babies are not drinking, they are not getting hind milk because they are not getting any milk. The baby in the above video came off the first breast *drinking* and did not want the second side. Many mothers will keep the baby on the first side until the baby has nibbled himself to sleep (like on a pacifier). This emphasis on feeding one breast at a feeding, sometimes even several feedings in a row on the same breast ("block feeding") so the baby gets the "hind milk" is discussed only to condemn this approach.

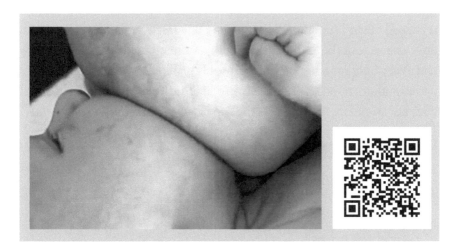

This 3-week-old drinks really well. The chin pause is longer and more sustained. Just like the previous baby, this baby is getting plenty of milk.

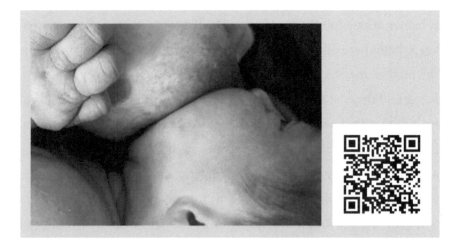

(This is the same video as the first one. It is shown again to emphasize the pause and the good asymmetric latch.)

## When Babies Do Not Drink Well

This 12-day-old baby in the video below is not drinking at all, though she is latched on and sucking. We cannot see *one single suck* where there is an obvious pause in the chin. This is nibbling rather than drinking. This baby had a very tight tongue-tie, which probably resulted in a dramatic decrease in the mother's milk supply and flow. Tongue-tie leads to a poor latch, which does not stimulate the mother's milk to be adequately released.

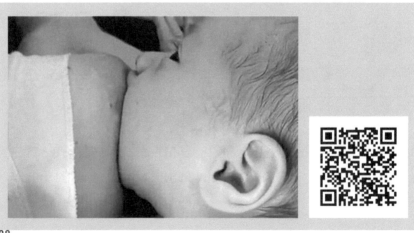

It's amazing that after 12 days of this type of feeding that the baby is not seriously dehydrated, yet she was not. Likely the mother's flow of milk *was* adequate at first, but her milk supply decreased. To reiterate, the chin pause tells us when the baby is receiving milk. Longer pauses mean more milk flow. Timed feedings make no sense. A baby drinking *well* for 10 minutes will get a lot more milk than one who spends an hour sucking on the breast with little or no milk flow at all.

This 8-week-old baby is also hardly drinking. Apparently, everything was going well until the baby was 6 weeks old. At the 6-week postpartum visit to her doctor, the mother was prescribed a combination birth control pill and her milk supply dropped dramatically. It does not take long for the hormones in the birth control pill to decrease milk supply. It may happen within a week.

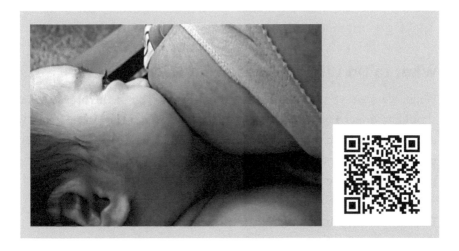

Sometimes the baby is "in between" getting lots of milk or getting virtually none, or the drinking is described as "borderline," as you can see in this video.

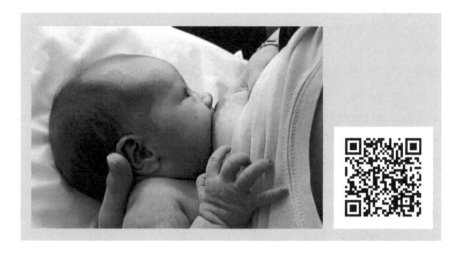

This baby is 2 weeks old and *apparently* below birthweight. Birthweight was measured in hospital and the 2-week weight was measured in the doctor's office on a different scale. One thing was clear: the baby was drinking poorly much of the time, with few chin pauses. So what did we do?

## What to Do When Babies Are Not Drinking Well

When we observe that babies are not drinking well at the breast, what should be done? First of all, adjust the latch so that it they have a goodly amount of breast in their mouths and the latch is asymmetric as discussed earlier in this chapter. With a good latch, mothers are less likely to have pain and babies are likely to receive more milk from the breast.

### Teach Mothers to Know When Babies Are Drinking Well

We should then teach mothers how to tell if their babies are *drinking* while on the breast. This is *vital*. Health professionals, particularly pediatricians, may believe that babies are getting milk if the breast in their mouths and they make sucking movements, but it isn't necessarily so. If babies are not gaining well, health professionals may assume that it is problem with the milk itself rather than a problem of the baby not getting the milk that is available.

## Use Breast Compressions

We teach mothers to use breast compressions. When the baby's sucking slows and they start nibbling, the mother compresses her breast to increase the flow of milk. When the flow slows even with compression, mothers release the compression. Breast compressions are essentially like pumping, but the milk goes directly into the baby not into a plastic or glass receptacle. See this video in a 2-day-old baby responding to the use of breast compression.

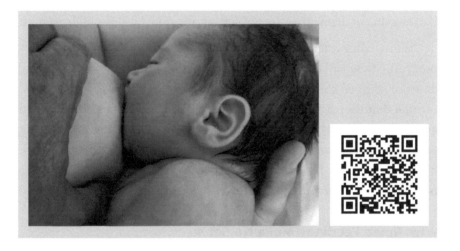

I (JN) am doing the compressions to show the mother the technique. Here is another video showing breast compressions in a 4-day-old.

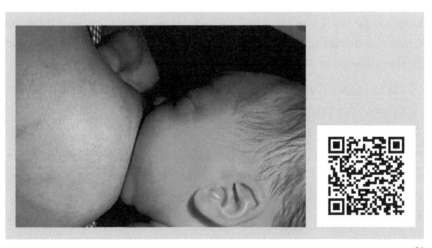

## Offer the Other Breast

When babies no longer drink even with compressions, we recommend that mothers then offer the other breast before babies becomes too sleepy. If the baby was drinking as was the 3-week-old, who at first was not latching on, the baby might not take the second breast—or he might. Many health professionals tell mothers to only use one breast to ensure that the baby gets more high-fat hind milk. The longer a baby drinks, the higher the concentration fat in the milk. The key phrase is *the longer the baby drinks*. If babies do not drink, they are not getting any milk let alone high-fat milk.

Young babies sleeping at the breast does not necessarily mean they are "full." They will often sleep at the breast because milk flow is slowing down or stopped completely. Mothers see that their babies are asleep and assume that they have had enough. They take their babies off the breast and within minutes, many babies show they are still hungry by rooting, and may quickly start to cry. Parents and doctors may assume that their babies are fussy or have colic or allergies to something in the mother's milk (cows'-milk protein, for example).

## Why Timed Feedings Make No Sense

Some health professionals still tell mothers to feed the baby for, say, 10 minutes on each side. Of course, this makes no sense. A baby who is drinking very little at the breast can spend a long time on the breast without receiving much milk. Babies do not feed by the clock and their internal clock says, "keep eating until you have had enough." This idea of feeding the baby X minutes on each breast is based on bottle-feeding norms. It takes the average baby 20 to 30 minutes to finish a bottle.

As milk flow slows, younger babies may fall asleep, while older babies pull away from the breast. In neither case does it mean, necessarily, that the baby has had enough milk.

Timed feedings do not make sense for another reason; mothers do not necessarily produce equal amounts of milk in both breasts. Babies may also prefer one side to the other, often because the latch is better on the preferred side, thus unequally stimulating milk production. Or the baby always received more milk from one breast than the other, right from the beginning of breastfeeding. The body is not 100% symmetric, and thus the right breast may produce more milk than the left, or vice versa.

## Conclusion

This chapter summarizes the key aspects of breastfeeding management that we use in our practice. Observing babies at the breast, making sure that babies are latched on well and are drinking well from the breast, are essential parts of lactation support. Furthermore, it is important to emphasize that breastfeeding should not hurt. When babies are not drinking well, mothers should use breast compressions and always offer the other breast. Mothers and babies may need additional support, but this is something that everyone who works with breastfeeding mothers should know.

## CHAPTER 11

# Breast Pain, Infection, and Lumps

As is true with nipple pain, breast pain means that there is something wrong. Ideally, mothers should get breastfeeding support immediately after birth, and then as often as necessary, to make sure the baby is latched on and *drinking well*. This is rarely done, unfortunately. The mother gets attention only if there are problems, often times, not even then. Too often the "attention" involves giving the baby bottles or someone offering the mother a nipple shield. Unfortunately, this type of "help" too often leads to breastfeeding failure. When breastfeeding fails, it is not the mother's fault. We blame the healthcare system and its inability to help effectively. Health professionals need good information; information they have never received in their training or experience. Below are some common types of breast pain and what can be done to help.

## Engorgement

Many health professionals believe it is normal for the mother's breast to be engorged when the milk "comes in" at 3 or 4 days after birth. They may even think that engorgement is good because it means that the mother will produce lots of milk. We argue that engorgement is neither normal nor good. If babies are breastfeeding well from birth, and have not received bottles or pacifiers, mothers may feel *slightly* full at 3 or 4 days, but they should not be in pain from engorgement. (To repeat for emphasis, any fullness should not be painful.) Conversely, the absence of significant engorgement is not worrisome. What matters is that the baby is drinking well and the mother is not having nipple or breast pain.

Babies not latching on well and drinking poorly at the breast is the main reason why mothers get painfully engorged. Mothers need good breastfeeding help from the start to ensure a good latch which prevents painful engorgement as well as so many other breastfeeding problems.

## Other Causes of Painful Engorgement

Besides a poor latch and baby not drinking well from the breast, there are other factors that lead to engorgement.

### Intravenous Fluids

Fluids mothers receive during labor contribute to painful engorgement. Fluids tend to go to the areas of the body with the greatest blood supply, such as the breasts. Synthetic oxytocin (Pitocin) also causes fluid retention.

Pumping the breasts probably won't help with engorgement, it can make it worse as the pump may pull fluid to the front of the breast, without getting much milk, and could give mothers the impression that they are not producing any milk. Why not just get the baby latched on well? If it is difficult to latch the baby on, then initiate reverse-pressure softening of the nipple and areola as shown in the video.

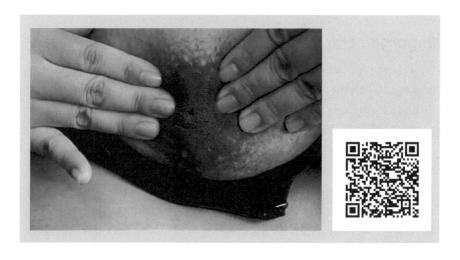

If the baby still does not latch on well, mothers can hand express and feed their milk to their babies using a cup or lactation aid at the breast.

## Blocked Ducts and Mastitis

Blocked ducts and mastitis are also a consequence of babies not latching on well. Mothers may develop fever, body aches and pains, chills, and sweating, but they don't always. Blocked ducts and mastitis can resolve spontaneously, without antibiotics, but sometimes, antibiotics are necessary. Let's not forget to help the baby with a better, more effective latch which probably would have prevented the blocked ducts or mastitis in the first place.

As with everything in medicine, *prevention* is better than treatment. Prevention means ensuring that the baby has a good latch as soon as possible after birth. We frequently find that babies also have a tongue-tie, which prevents a good latch. The tongue-tie does not have to be severe to result in poor drainage of the breast.

### Blocked Ducts

Blocked ducts can be caused by a poor latch, which leads to poor breast drainage. If the mother's milk supply is abundant, babies will sometimes get milk well no matter how bad the latch is, *up to a point*. As time passes, a poor latch means that the mother may remain engorged or "full" even after the baby has finished drinking. Remaining engorged or even feeling full after a feeding is not a good sign, though many mothers will take this as a sign they have plenty of milk. Perhaps they do, but the breasts should not remain obviously full. When the breast is only partially emptied, it compresses other parts and prevents those parts of the breast from emptying well. Thus, an area of blockage remains, which may become infected with the result the mother develops mastitis and on occasion may go on to abscess formation.

Lactation consultants often tell mothers who are engorged a lot of the time that they have an "oversupply" of milk. We believe that oversupply of milk is extremely over-diagnosed (see Chapter 24), Myths Even Many

Lactation Consultants Believe). If the mother's breast is still full after a feeding, it means the baby was not latched on well, and the breast is not draining well. Mothers with abundant milk supplies are also often encouraged to feed the baby on only one breast at a feeding. This can cause engorgement in the other breast, possible blocking ducts and decreasing milk supply and flow over time.

## Mastitis

Mastitis is an infection of an area of the breast with poor drainage. Antibiotics are not always necessary since mastitis often gets better without specific treatment *if the mother continues breastfeeding.* We recommend improving the latch and continuing breastfeeding on the affected side allowing the infection to take its course over 12 to 24 hours. If the mastitis improves by 12 to 18 hours, antibiotics may not be necessary. If antibiotics are started, then the mother should start feeling better within 12 hours, and definitely within 24 hours, though it may take a few days for her to feel 100% better.

Many doctors prescribe antibiotics when the mother has pain in the breast, even if there are no signs of infection (swelling, redness, and pain in a part of the breast often associated with the mother having fever). We believe this is inappropriate. Pain in the breast without signs of infection is not an indication to start antibiotics. In general, if mothers have had symptoms of mastitis for less than 24 hours, we recommend waiting on starting antibiotics. However, we also remain alert to possible very rapid worsening of the pain, swelling, fever, malaise. Luckily this does not occur often. We recently had one breastfeeding mother who went from "blocked duct" to full blown mastitis in less than 8 hours. We have only seen such a case once over the years.

Many bacterial infections improve spontaneously without antibiotics. Of course, not treating a bacterial infection requires careful monitoring of the patient's condition. Unfortunately, some health professionals find it much easier to treat and make a relieved sigh as they will no longer need to worry about the patient. Unfortunately, antibiotics can cause significant problems and on rare occasions, even death. If they can be avoided, that is a good thing. We must remember too that because of overuse of antibiotics, some bacteria are now resistant to all the antibiotics currently available.

If antibiotics are required, we do not recommend amoxicillin, which, for some bizarre reason is frequently prescribed for mastitis in Southern Ontario. In our experience, *Staphylococcus aureus* is the most common infecting agent by far and is *not* sensitive to amoxicillin. That "mastitis" frequently gets better when the mother takes amoxicillin suggests that either she did not have mastitis, or, that if she did have mastitis, it proves that mastitis can get better without antibiotic treatment. In our practice, we choose cotrimoxazole, which is made up of sulfamethoxazole and trimethoprim. These two antibiotics reduce the chances that the *Staphylococcus* is resistant or will become resistant.

After the infection is controlled, it is time to go back to the basics: make sure the breast is well drained with every feed, improving the baby's latch, using breast compression, and offering both breasts at each feeding.

Heat packs applied to the swollen area can help the mother's body fight off infection (Evans, Repasky, & Fisher, 2015). Heat mobilizes anti-infective molecules in one's body, which is why the body develops fever when someone has an infection. In fact, a low temperature in a sick baby with an infection is not a good prognostic sign. In general, it is better not to bring down a fever unless one feels terrible with it. Note, however, that often, young children are quite comfortable with fever, even high fever, unlike older children and adults.

## Breast Abscess

Abscesses are a result of our bodies trying to wall off an infection and prevent septicemia (a generalized blood infection), which can be fatal, so in a way, an abscess can be a good thing. Abscesses are generally painful and usually develop because of delayed or inadequate treatment of mastitis. Abscesses sometimes develop because practitioners tell mothers not to breastfeed on a breast with mastitis. The best way to decrease risk of abscess is to continue draining the breast.

We diagnose abscesses based on clinical suspicion (history, palpation of a lump that contains liquid), and then by aspiration of the lump as in the photo below. Aspiration of pus makes the diagnosis. We aspirate pus for several reasons.

1.   Removing as much of the pus as practical will give the mother some pain relief, at least temporarily until the pus re-accumulates.

2.   The presence of pus confirms diagnosis.

3.   The pus can be sent for culture and sensitivity to antibiotics immediately until definitive treatment can be arranged.

The syringe in the photo below contains pus, but the milk at the end of the nipple looks normal. It is possible that the abscess will burst into a milk duct, but we have not seen that happen in more than 150 mothers with breast abscess that we have seen in our clinic. For this reason, and to prevent engorgement, mothers should continue to breastfeed on the affected side.

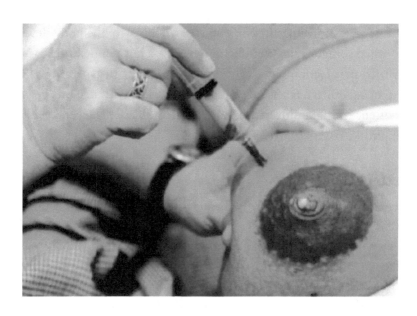

## Who Should Treat a Breast Abscess?

We do not usually send mothers to see a surgeon, even a specialized breast surgeon. In our experience, surgeons, as a group, tend not to support breast-feeding. There are always exceptions, of course. Many surgeons support breastfeeding but they often still give mothers bad advice. For example, they may tell mothers that they must completely stop breastfeeding, thinking that they need to "dry up" or the abscess will not heal. How do they *not* know that continued breastfeeding on one side does *not* stimulate milk production on the other? In other words, a mother can, if necessary, dry up on one side and continue breastfeeding on the other. However, drying up the milk, even in the breast with an abscess, is neither necessary or desirable.

A breast abscess is also not a dire emergency. Definitive drainage does not have to be done in the emergency department in the middle of the night. Too often, surgeons or emergency physicians drain abscesses without taking breastfeeding into consideration. For example, the location of incisions can make a huge difference. See the photo below. This mother's obstetrician diagnosed the abscess by history and physical examination. The mother, on the advice of her obstetrician, told the surgeon not to do a periareolar incision to drain the abscess, but the surgeon did a periare-olar incision anyway. This is unconscionable arrogance on the part of the surgeon and did not consider the needs of the mother and baby at all.

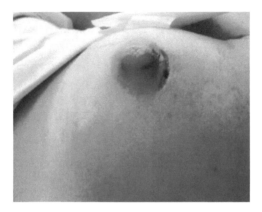

In this case, the periareolar incision resulted in several problems for the mother.

1.  **Pain.** As with any incision anywhere on the body, pain from this incision will be severe enough that most mothers will not put the baby to that breast. This can lead to the breast producing less milk because the mother cannot easily empty her breast to maintain the supply. Even expressing by hand would be awkward and painful.

2.  **Engorgement.** The mother is likely to become engorged on that side because she is unlikely to be able to breastfeed or express her milk without pain.

3.  **Severed Milk Ducts.** This incision would likely have cut several milk ducts.

4.  **Increased Risk of a Milk Fistula.** Milk will continue to drain from that side and the mother cannot breastfeed or express because of pain.

5.  **Possible Future Low Milk Supply.** Although we do not know for sure that periareolar incisions diminish future breastmilk production, we frequently see evidence of this in our clinic patients. The longer the incision, the higher the chance that breastmilk production will be affected. We have never done a formal study, but we have seen this problem over and over again.

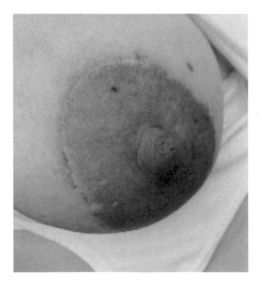

In the above photo, the mother had this periareolar incision for an open biopsy and the baby drank much less on this breast compared to the other. Coincidence? We do not think so. We do not understand why the surgeon used an incision like this for an open biopsy. This sort of incision (though it is usually done all around the areola) is more common with breast reduction surgery, but it is doubtful the mother needed such an incision for a biopsy. Surgeons, if at all possible, should keep incisions on the breast as far away from the nipple and areola.

The next photo shows the breast of a mother who had surgery for an abscess 2 years before this photo. She was seen at our clinic when she was pregnant again because she wanted to know if the surgery would affect her ability to breastfeed the new baby.

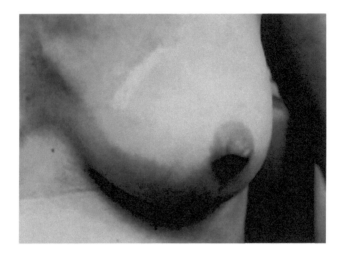

The answer? Probably not. However, this incision, though far from the nipple and areola was done in such a way that the incision will likely tend to remain open by the weight of the breast and thus healing could be delayed. Also, it was likely that more breast ducts would be cut, unless the abscess was very close to the skin. An incision perpendicular to that scar would not have compromised the drainage of the breast, while at the same time would have avoided the above-mentioned problems. It should be said that this is a very large incision to drain a breast abscess.

## Here Is a Better Way of Treating an Abscess

Ulitzsch and colleagues (2004) describe a method of draining an abscess that is more likely to preserve breast function in the short- and long-term, while allowing the mother to continue breastfeeding on the breast with the abscess. Unfortunately, the article was published in a radiology journal, so most surgeons probably haven't seen it.

How does this technique work? First of all, it is done by intervention radiologists, not surgeons. The radiologist maps out the abscess using ultrasound, making sure to see if the abscess is multi-locular or a single abscess. Then a catheter is inserted, as far from the nipple and areola as is practical. The drain stays in place (see photo below) until there is no more drainage and then the drain is removed, either at once, or some radiologists withdraw it slowly over a few days. The mother continues breastfeeding normally on both breasts throughout the treatment.

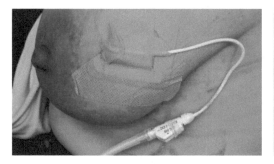 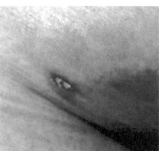

The photo on the left shows the catheter in place. Note that the mother can continue breastfeeding. The photo on the right shows where the catheter was placed and then taken out about 7 to 10 days later (it was withdrawn slowly). (The second photo is not the breast of the mother in the first photo to the left.)

## Galactocele

A galactocele is a collection of milk, surrounded by a membrane, located in the breast. It seems to develop in a previous blocked duct. Sometimes it can enlarge dramatically and, as it enlarges, it will usually cause the mother pain, depending on how quickly it enlarges. However, once the pressure of the liquid in the galactocele equals the pressure in the breast surrounding it, the mother's pain usually stops as the galactocele should not continue to expand.

We aspirate a fluid-filled lump in the breast, once only, to make the diagnosis, because ultrasound, a common diagnostic approach to a mass in the breast, does not reliably distinguish between types of fluid in the galactocele. Thus, the fluid could be milk, in which case, it is a galactocele. If it is pus, it is an abscess. The fluid could also contain malignant cells, though the latter is quite unusual in our practice, thankfully.

Too often, however, breastfeeding mothers are subjected to repeated aspirations in the vain hope of curing the galactocele. From our experience with many mothers with galactoceles, this is not a useful approach. The galactocele almost always just refills after each aspiration, often within a few hours. With each aspiration, there is a risk of infecting the fluid. Here is a typical story our clinic received by email.

> At 4 weeks postpartum I was diagnosed with a very large and painful galactocele in my left breast. I had this drained twice. When it refilled, it had pus in it and was then diagnosed as an abscess, which I had drained a further two times.
>
> It then refilled and created channels in my breast (authors' note: not sure what "channels in my breast" means), and a couple of weeks ago it burst. I've been having the wound packed, and it is healing very well. I have continued to exclusively breastfeed only from my right breast as it became impossible to feed from the left. I do still have a small amount of milk coming from the left. My concern is, if I start to express or feed from the left, will stimulating my milk cause the galactocele/abscess to fill back up? Or is that not likely now that it has burst and is healing from the inside out?

Thus, this mother had two drainages of the galactocele, which we would argue is one too many. The second aspiration likely introduced infection and the galactocele became an abscess.

Galactoceles are very difficult to deal with if the mother has significant pain. Nevertheless, treatment with analgesics can be helpful until the galactocele reaches the size where it no longer causes pain.

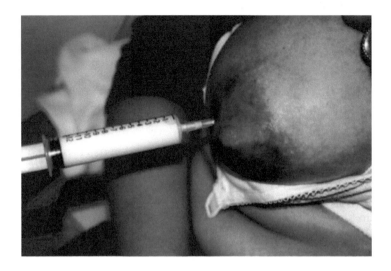

The above photo shows the aspiration of a galactocele. The mother had no pain but was concerned about what this swelling she felt in her breast. After diagnosis, we asked her to watch for signs of infection (pain, redness of the overlying area). Breast abscess is not necessarily associated with fever, though a preceding mastitis often is.

The best way to deal with a galactocele after diagnosis is to leave it alone. The mother should continue breastfeeding as long as she and the baby desire, but once the mother has stopped breastfeeding and the milk "dried up," *if* the galactocele is still present, a single aspiration will likely cure it. If it does not resolve once the mother stops breastfeeding, and drainage by aspiration does not cure it, there are surgical procedures that can cure a galactocele, but these are very rarely necessary. Note that we are not recommending stopping breastfeeding for the presence of a galactocele. It would also be a good idea too avoid any sort of surgery on the breast when a mother is breastfeeding if possible.

## Investigating a Lump in the Breast

Some mothers develop a lump in the breast and the question comes up: could it be cancer? Women who breastfeed have a proven lower risk of breast cancer, and the longer they breastfed the lower the risk (Collaborative Group on Hormonal Factors in Breast Cancer, 2002). Unfortunately, breastfeeding does not provide 100% protection against anything. Some breastfeeding women do develop breast cancer. A few develop it even while they are still breastfeeding. Also unfortunately, the investigation of a breast lump often undermines breastfeeding.

The mother in the photo below had an *emergency* ultrasound of the lump in her armpit. The photo was taken in our clinic when the baby was 2 weeks old.

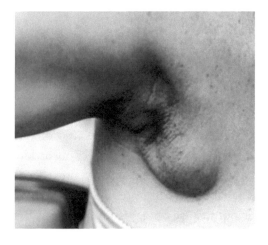

What *is* this? Answer: Normal breast tissue in the mother's armpit. Such swellings are common. In our clinic, we see such a swelling at least once a day. The lump decreases in size over time. Yet instead of waiting for the lump to disappear normally over a few weeks, this mother received an unnecessary test, as an emergency, perhaps displacing a more urgent case from having an ultrasound. The fact that the lump decreased in size the entire time was very reassuring, no? Below, another example, showing not only a lump, but also a nipple that leaks milk.

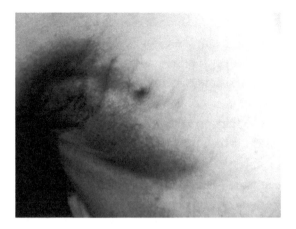

Here is a story that we hear, with variations, not infrequently.

Two lumps were found in my breast during my pregnancy, and it was recommended I get them biopsied. I got the core biopsy done at 10 days postpartum. I have had constant milk leakage from the incision site (6 days now). Yesterday I soaked through 4 hospital maxi pads. I went to the doctor today and was told that the lumps were benign fibroadenomas, and to wait 1 week to see if the leaking stops, and if it doesn't, I'll need to stop breastfeeding altogether. She said if I wait longer, I'm at high risk for infection and mastitis. I don't want to stop breastfeeding, and I'm wondering how often milk duct fistulas heal on their own. Just want your opinion and what you recommend.

There is so much wrong with what happened to this mother. First of all, if it were important to rule out breast cancer, then why not do a biopsy during pregnancy? Clearly the doctor did not think an aggressive breast cancer was likely if she was willing to wait months to make a diagnosis. Considering the mother's problems after the core biopsy, these problems could have been avoided if the biopsy had been done during pregnancy when the amount of milk in the breast was low. Doing the biopsy while she was breastfeeding was much more likely to cause problems.

The doctor also gave her fanciful advice. True, the mother may develop a fistula, but 2 weeks after the biopsy is not a long enough time to wait to see if the leaking would stop on its own. We have seen leaking stop even one month after a biopsy. Is there anything that could be done to stop the leaking? We would suggest skin glue of the incision site plus staples to close the incision. If it is difficult for milk to exit the incision site, will it not find its way to the normal exit? Maybe not, and a galactocele might develop at the site. Or the milk might break through the incision despite skin glue and staples. Given the problems this mother encountered, it would have been worth a try to allow the mother to keep breastfeeding even on the affected side. It is possible that "blocking" the exit from the incision site while continuing breastfeeding may have worked. We suggest that a galactocele may be preferable to constant leaking.

The mother could stop breastfeeding if nothing is helping, but *only* on the side of the biopsy. Clearly the surgeon never even considered this possibility. She probably believes that if the mother continues breastfeeding on the other breast, milk production will continue on the biopsied side, which is simply not true. A mother can dry up on just one side. Continued breastfeeding on just one breast does not stimulate the other breast to continue producing milk. Most breast surgeons do not know this. If the mother continues leaking, stopping breastfeeding will not stop it. The lesson here is that a biopsy during pregnancy would have been less of a problem for the mother.

On the other hand, if a biopsy is not urgent, then why not approach the problem differently? An ultrasound of the lumps could indicate if they are not cancer. If the ultrasound is not definitive, then repeated ultrasounds done every couple of months might have been a better way of dealing with the problem. After all, the mother had already waited several months for the biopsy. Following the lumps with ultrasound may be reassuring. True, ultrasounds are not always good at defining what sort of a lump is present in the breast. But cancers grow, and if the lumps did not grow, they are unlikely to be cancer. Furthermore, the surgeon told the mother that if leaking did not stop in a week there was a strong chance of developing an infection or mastitis, which is probably not true either. Leaking nipples do not increase the chances of mastitis. Mastitis is due to infection of a poorly drained area of the breast.

This, by the way, we frequently hear variations of this problem. Some surgeons dive into recommending a biopsy when other approaches would not cause problems for the breastfeeding mother and baby (how inconvenient is it to soak four hospital maxi-pads?).

This picture shows a breast abscess that developed after a breast biopsy. Is it too much to suggest that biopsies of the breast should not be taken lightly?

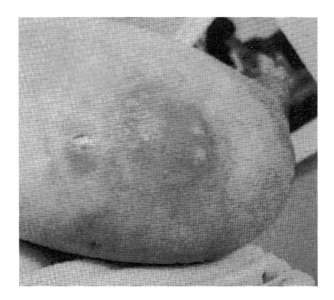

## Conclusion

As is true with nipple pain, breast pain is not normal and is a signal that something is wrong. Engorgement, blocked ducts, and mastitis are signs that babies are not drinking well at the breast. Lumps can be galactoceles, abscesses, or more rarely, cancer. They need to be assessed and possibly treated, preferably by practitioners who know about and care about breastfeeding. Lumps under the arm should also be assessed, but can be normal breast tissue, which will go away on its own.

# CHAPTER 12

# Tongue-Tie

By definition, a baby with a tongue-tie has a less than ideal latch. A tongue-tie can also cause late onset decreasing milk supply and flow, as can any cause of a poor latch. Unfortunately, many pediatricians and nurses do not believe that tongue-tie causes breastfeeding problems and/or do not know how to diagnose a tongue-tie. Even when health professionals know about tongue-ties, parents are often the ones who find them.

Tongue-ties may cause a range of breastfeeding problems. Babies with severe tongue-ties may have difficulty eating food. The tongue-tie makes it hard to move food from the front to the back of their mouths so the baby can swallow the food easily. Tongue-ties can make it hard to pronounce certain words or produce a "rolled" r, which is common in many languages including Spanish, Arabic, some languages from India, and Slavic languages.

British midwives in the early 20th century knew about tongue-ties. We have heard that they grew a long baby fingernail to release tongue-ties in newborns in the first days of life. We believe that health professionals stopped considering tongue-tie an issue when breastfeeding rates plummeted; when it was no longer the norm to breastfeed, and our society forgot how breastfeeding works. Many health professionals look at tongue-ties in much the same way as tonsillectomy—basically a fad, which is a real issue for an occasional baby or child, but only very occasionally.

Our combined experience of 55 years working with mothers and babies with breastfeeding problems, and at least 40 years of combined experience with releasing tongue-ties, supports our belief that tongue-tie has negative effects on breastfeeding success. Typically, we diagnose three, four, or more babies with tongue-tie in a single day. (Obviously, at a breastfeeding clinic, we collect breastfeeding problems.) Tongue-tie causes significant difficulties with breastfeeding, in the form of problems latching on, mothers having sore nipples, babies who do not get enough from the breast, and babies who refuse the breast because the flow of milk is slow. Release of tongue-ties often results in *immediate* and sustained improvement of the breastfeeding problems, particularly if the release is done soon after the baby's birth (within 1 to 2 weeks, and even better on the first day or two of life).

Oddly, some healthcare providers insist that tongue-ties *cannot* interfere with breastfeeding. At least three hospitals in the Toronto area now forbid healthcare professionals from speaking to new parents about tongue-tie. We have heard similar stories from other countries. Parents tell us that no one even bothered looking into the baby's mouth. Indeed, in our clinic, we have identified many cases of tongue-tie and have even picked up *three* missed cases of cleft palate in one single year, which suggests strongly that nobody is looking in the baby's mouth. Indeed, now that postpartum physical examinations are done in the presence of the family, we believe them. Fair enough, the parents may not have noticed, but when we ask, it is rare that they noticed the doctor checking inside the baby's mouth.

## Tongue-Tie Alone May Not Be a Problem

So why has tongue-tie "suddenly" become a bigger and bigger problem over the past 30 or 40 years? We believe that this "epidemic" has occurred because, unless extremely tight, tongue-ties did not always cause the problems that they do today. Tongue-tie *alone may not be the problem a lot of the time.* It is the combination of the negative effects on breastfeeding that begin with labor and birth (see Chapter 6). After an ideal birth, a tongue-tie alone might not cause significant problems. However, combine the presence of a tongue-tie with the interventions around labor, birth, and the immediate postpartum period and suddenly, what might not have been a problem becomes a considerable problem. Indeed, we occasionally see a mother and baby in the clinic who are having no problems at all with breastfeeding, at least not at the time we see them, about 2 or 3 weeks after the birth, the tongue-tie noted themselves, or by a friend or by a midwife, but not a physician, usually. We used to leave the decision of whether or not to release the tongue-tie to the parents, suggesting that they watch out for signs of late onset decreased milk supply and flow. However, we believe now that the tongue-tie should be released to prevent late onset decreased milk supply and flow. (See Chapter 15)

## An Anecdote

When we tell parents that their baby has a tongue-tie, a long discussion typically ensues, often because healthcare providers told them that there was no tongue-tie or that it wouldn't make any difference for breastfeeding. They worry about releasing a tongue-tie if it does not make a difference.

One day, we saw a family at the clinic originally from Serbia. The mother had severe sore nipples. After the history was taken, and I (JN) examined the baby, I told the parents that the baby had a tongue-tie and that this was a likely cause of the mother's nipple pain. The father immediately said, "cut it." I was surprised because usually there is a 20- to 30-minute discussion including, "Do you think this is what causes my pain?" "Does it need to be released right away?" "Could the pain be due to something else?" In any case, we released the tongue-tie. After it was done, I asked the father why he was so willing, without any discussion, to have the tongue-tie released. The father answered that he had had a tongue-tie as a child, and he was unable to properly pronounce certain words in Serbian. Other children viciously mocked him at school. When he was 25, he finally had his tongue-tie released and could finally pronounce Serbian the same way everyone else did. He did not want his child to have the same problem.

Another Serbian couple told me that in the countryside in Serbia, every newborn baby gets a tongue-tie release at birth. They use a sugar cube to do the release (a simple push on the frenulum with an index finger would do the trick as well if the baby is only a day or two old). As studies have shown, a little sugar does seem to work as a temporary "anesthetic" in newborns but breastfeeding before and after the procedure also works very well.

## Diagnosing Tongue-Tie

The frenulum is tight if it limits the tongue's *upward* movement. In severe cases, it is almost impossible to get our fingers under the tongue. In tongues with questionably tight frenula, we diagnose tongue-tie based on mothers' and babies' symptoms. Breastfeeding should not be painful for the mother. Babies should be able to latch on and receive milk well from the breast. We will release a "borderline" tongue-tie if breastfeeding is painful, or the baby is not latching on or drinking from the breast.

### Sore Nipples and Decreased Milk Supply and Flow

Tongue-tie interferes with how the baby latches on, often resulting in sore nipples for the mother and the baby's decreased milk intake. Problems usually appear immediately after birth. It is not uncommon that mothers may overcome the early difficulties but then develop late onset sore nipples. In our experience, late onset decreasing milk supply often causes late onset sore nipples. There are two possible reasons for a new onset of sore nipples. First, babies may pull on the breast without letting go, which causes pain and damage.

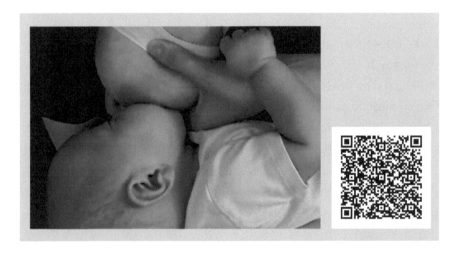

Babies may also slip down on the nipple when the milk flow slows and they no longer have a good latch. Nipple pain should be taken seriously, even if—especially if—it starts after several weeks. The return of the mother's menstrual period can occur as early as 3 months after birth and can be a symptom of decreasing milk supply. The return of menses does not decrease milk supply, as is frequently thought. Rather, mothers' decreased milk supply and flow caused mother's menses to return. New-onset sore nipples can also be a sign of a new pregnancy for many women, which will reduce milk supply.

We do not know how many mothers of babies with significant tongue-ties end up with late- onset decreasing milk supply and flow. We do not see them in our clinic unless there is a recognized breastfeeding problem. Too often, however, we observe that babies were misdiagnosed with colic or allergy, and treatment is delayed. We doubt that exclusively breastfed babies are allergic to milk or have reflux. According to Munblit and colleagues (2020):

> Recommendations to manage common infant symptoms as CMA (cow-milk allergy) are not evidence-based, especially in breastfed infants who are not directly consuming cow milk. Such recommendations may cause harm by undermining confidence in breastfeeding (p. 599).

## "Significant" Tongue-Tie

Many physical signs have been used to define significantly tight lingual frenula. A significant tongue-tie restricts the upward mobility of the tongue. Pediatricians often assume that if babies can stick out their tongues that there is no tie. Unfortunately, sticking out a tongue does not rule tongue-tie out. A heart-shaped tongue suggests a significant tongue-tie, which restricts the *upward* motion of the tongue.

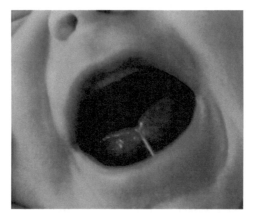

In this photo, the baby is crying. Normally, the tongue would lift higher, closer to the palate. The tongue is also heart shaped. This baby's tongue-tie is significantly restricting the movement of the tongue.

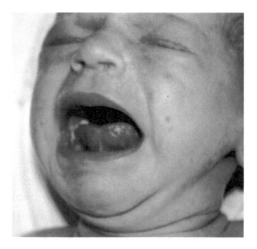

This baby also has vertical restriction of the tongue, and, incidentally, he also has thrush. It is important to mention the thrush since many babies with tongue-tie have a white "milky" tongue, which is frequently misdiagnosed as thrush. Thrush occurs on the inside of the cheeks, sometimes on the palate and occasionally on the gums. If "whiteness" is only on the tongue, it is not thrush. A white tongue only is associated with tongue-tie.

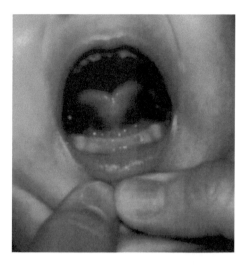

This baby's tongue (above photo) shows definite restriction of the vertical movement with the typical heart shape. Yet, no frenulum is obvious. Restriction of vertical tongue movement is the real diagnostic feature of a tongue-tie.

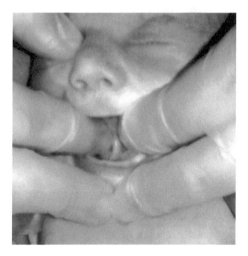

This is another tongue-tie that is not obvious by just looking at the mouth but becomes obvious in trying to lift the tongue. Breastfeeding improved when the tongue-tie was released.

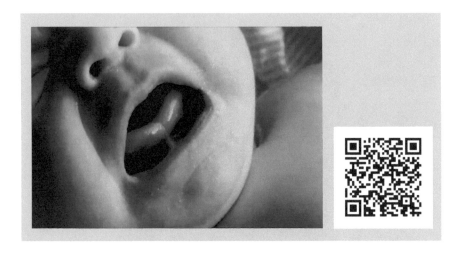

It is clear in this video that the baby's tongue movement is restricted.

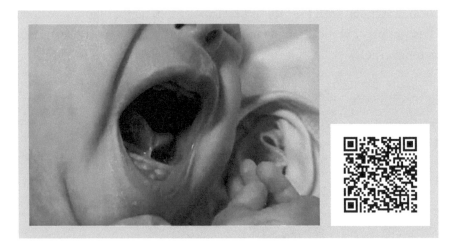

These videos are remarkable because the parents and babies were seen at our clinic on the same day. Furthermore, each was seen by a different pediatrician who would *usually* have done a tongue-tie release, but both refused because the babies were latching on and gaining weight. However, both mothers had significant, even disabling, pain.

These two pediatricians, and their lack of response to the mothers' pain, highlight a real problem in our health system. Pediatricians take care of babies, so, if babies are latching on and gaining well, mothers' pain is not the pediatrician's problem. Obstetricians take care of mothers, right? However, once the baby is born, unless there is a problem attributable to the birth, obstetricians are not in the picture at all.

## Releasing Tongue-Ties

Until recently, we did not want to release tongue-ties if there were no apparent problems. We have changed our minds because tongue-tie can cause late onset decreasing milk supply 6 weeks to 4 months after birth. Late onset decreasing milk supply can happen as early as 3 or 4 weeks. We believe in releasing tongue-ties as soon as possible after birth. If mothers do not want to have the release done right away, we tell them to watch for signs of decreased milk supply and flow and to get help at the first sign of trouble. Still, it is better to release early and prevent problems in the first place.

### How We Do a Tongue-Tie Release

In our clinic, we immobilize the baby, while a lactation consultant shines a bright light on the baby's mouth, avoiding shining the light into the baby's eyes. I (JN) snip about a millimeter of the frenulum, and then push on the cut with the index finger of my left hand until I can push no more. The frenulum is released with very *little* pressure and takes only a second. If the frenulum had not been released before, it is usually thin and tears easily. The result is a diamond shaped wound. Bleeding occurs only occasionally, or it oozes for a couple of seconds. When mothers put babies to the breast immediately after the procedure, it almost always stops bleeding. Generally, we ask parents to stay in the room for the procedure so that the baby can go straight to the breast. We do not use any anesthetic as breastfeeding is the best anesthetic. This is a video of the procedure. Note that it is in slow motion, and so the sound is distorted.

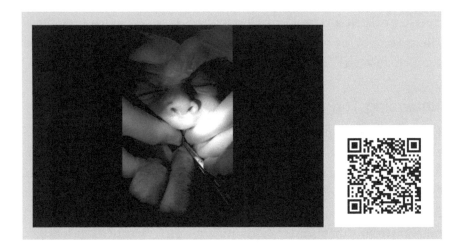

We recently (August 2021) had a baby whose bleeding lasted a couple of hours. I suspect that there was an aberrant blood vessel running along the edge of the frenulum. We put pressure on the wound with epinephrine-soaked gauze, which slowed the bleeding down. We also tried a silver nitrate stick. Neither stopped the bleeding, but the oozing was minimal and stopped on its own. I (JN) have had only two or three such babies out of thousands of babies whose frenulum was released.

## Laser Release of Tongue-Ties

Some dentists use lasers to do tongue-tie releases. We do not think that lasers work better than scissors. When I have watched laser releases, the baby seemed to be in pain during the entire procedure. The procedure takes more time than a scissors release and the baby cried the whole time. We have seen babies in our clinic who have had laser releases, but there was significant re-attachment regardless. All of this makes it difficult to know which procedure is best. Breastfeeding problems are only occasionally due to tongue-tie alone. If dentists do the procedure, they usually do not address other issues that may be causing problems (how to latch a baby on, how to know a baby is drinking at the breast, etc).

## Re-Attachment

Re-attachment is the main problem after tongue-tie release. One clear symptom of reattachment is return of sore nipples. Typically, for 2 to 3 days, the mother may have complete relief from nipple pain, but then, 2 or 3 days after the release, the pain has returned. The issue is how to prevent re-attachment. There is no clear answer. Dentists, otolaryngologists, or physicians who do tongue-tie releases often recommend "stretches" after tongue-tie release. They recommend starting the stretches 2 or 3 days after the release and then continue several times a day for up to a month or longer. Many parents do not comply because their babies scream bloody murder with every stretch. Even when stretches are gentle (index fingers on either side of the frenulum with gentle lift of the tongue), babies loudly cry (and parents also). In our clinic, we have gone back and forth over the years with recommending stretches. At first, we did not recommend stretches or exercises. Then we tried an informal study, where some babies would have stretches, others did not. At present, we are back to stretches for all babies. However, we are not impressed by stretches preventing reattachment.

Our *impression* is that about 1 in 4 tongue-tie releases done in our clinic have a significant re-attachment when the baby comes back for a 1-week follow-up. However, we know that many parents do not continue with even "gentle" stretches before they give up with them because their babies are crying. The parents are often traumatized as much as the baby. If a tongue-tie does re-attach, we recommend a second release. Again, it is our *impression* that the second releases have a much lower rate of re-attachment than the first release.

Unfortunately, our impression does not really measure the effectiveness of this procedure. Nevertheless, when a tongue-tie is released within the first week after birth, re-attachment seems quite unusual.

## Tongue-Tie Release and Domperidone

Tongue-tie release and domperidone are two treatments with different objectives in the situation of late onset decreasing milk supply and flow. Tongue-tie release improves latch and domperidone increases the milk supply and flow, which often results in the baby being happier at the breast. Many mothers think that tongue-tie release alone will cures babies' problems, and so may refuse domperidone. On the other hand, some mothers will take the domperidone and refuse the tongue-tie release.

Releasing the tongue-tie stops the milk supply's progressive drop, but it won't usually bring it back up to what it was. Yes, helping with the latch, using breast compression, offering both breasts at each feed, if only one breast at a feed was habitually offered, may help increase the flow, but often not enough. We believe the domperidone is an important therapeutic measure when milk supply has dropped, and not just icing on the therapeutic cake.

### Breast Refusal Following Release

If the baby is older than 2 to 3 months of age, we recommend releasing tongue-ties at the second visit, especially if the baby is fussy at the breast. If milk supply and flow is relatively slow, babies may refuse the breast once the tongue-tie is released. Usually, breast refusal is temporary, lasting 6 to 8 hours, more than long enough to have a screaming baby. Sometimes, the breast refusal seems permanent, but our lactation consultants can almost always help the mother latch the baby on.

## What About Upper Lip Ties?

The evidence for upper lip ties causing problems with breastfeeding is much less definite than it is for tongue-tie. A thick lip tie may cause a midline diastema in the *permanent* upper incisors (see photo, though clearly this is still a young baby, probably between 6 and 12 months of age). Note notch in the baby's tongue suggesting a tongue-tie.

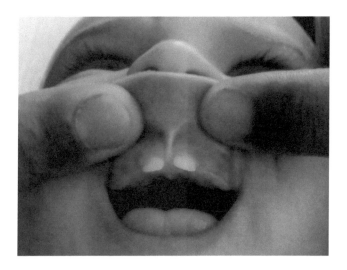

We've observed that if babies have a lip tie, they usually have a tongue-tie too. However, if babies have a tongue-tie, they do not necessarily also have a lip tie. The more pressing question is whether lip ties cause breastfeeding problems. We have seen no evidence that they do. The diagnostic criteria for lip tie are less clear than for a tongue-tie. Lactation consultants at our clinic suggest the following criteria for deciding if a lip tie is significant:

1. The mother has breast pain under the baby's upper lip.

2. The breast tissue proximal to the upper lip moves back and forth with each suck.

3. The upper lip does not flange out.

## Conclusion

Tongue-ties can cause significant problems with latching on to the breast and drinking well. They can also cause mothers significant amounts of pain. We recommend early release of tongue-ties, even in cases where they are borderline restricted as they may cause late onset decreasing milk supply and flow. One must also consider issues such as the mother's pain. There is much less evidence supporting release of lip ties as they do not seem to cause significant breastfeeding problems.

# CHAPTER 13

# Nipple Shields

Nipple shields are the bane of our existence. In our clinic, we often see 2 or 3 mothers *every day* who are feeding their babies through a nipple shield. Health professionals, including some lactation consultants, see nipple shields as the answer to all breastfeeding problems, from babies not latching on, to nipple soreness, to almost *routine* use in some hospitals for premature babies. What seems to be a quick fix for almost every possible breastfeeding problem, is nothing of the sort. Rather, nipple shields are more of an apparent fix, like "I don't know what to do, so try this."

## The Problem with Nipple Shields

If you are familiar with our work, you know that we strongly disagree with the use of nipple shields—ever. The real problem with the nipple shield is that the baby is *not* latched on to the breast. No matter how thin the nipple shield, it is still not the breast. Various health professionals recommend nipple shields for a wide range of problems but nipple shields rarely, if ever, fix the problem. Once a baby is "hooked" on the nipple shield, it becomes difficult to get the baby to take the breast. Indeed, a baby on a nipple shield is only *apparently* latched on, and thus, with time milk supply and the delivery of milk to the baby decreases, making it even more difficult to get the baby to take the breast directly. In our experience, the only mothers who manage with a nipple shield are those who have an *abundant* milk supply to start with. But then, with an abundant milk supply, the vast majority of their breastfeeding problems could have been, should have been, overcome without a nipple shield.

One mother in our practice had a first baby who refused breast. While still in the hospital, she was offered a nipple shield on *Day 2*. We really question this advice. If the baby was not latching on, it would have better to recommend the mother express her milk and cup feed her baby. *Even a bottle with expressed milk would have been better than a nipple shield.*

In this mother's case, the baby "breastfed" for 3 weeks but did not gain weight because her milk supply diminished: an expected result when feeding through a nipple shield. We saw the mother after her second baby because she had sore nipples but an abundance of milk at 4 weeks postpartum. Yes, some mothers produce more milk for one pregnancy versus another, but is it likely in this case? Is this a natural variation between two different breastfeeding experiences? Or did the nipple shields scuttle her supply for her first baby?

To repeat, we think nipple shields should be banned. They are a medical device that we should not recommend to mothers until research studies show that they actually help. To date, no such studies exist, and it is clear to the most casual of observers that they cause significant breastfeeding problems.

## Lowered Milk Supply

Nipple shields lower mothers' milk supply and flow of milk to the baby because the baby is not latching on directly on to the breast. The more milk supply diminishes, the harder it becomes to latch the baby on to the breast directly. One mother described her typical experience.

> I started using a breast shield when the baby was a few days old, after my milk came in... It seemed to go okay, but somewhere around 3 weeks I noticed she didn't seem to be sucking properly and by her one month check up she'd only gained an ounce (30 g).

Why start the nipple shield *after* the mother's milk "comes in"? Perhaps the mother's breasts were engorged, and the baby would not latch on. Or perhaps the baby never latched on and drank well in the first place. Another mother asked us this,

I started to pump from the second week because she was *not getting enough milk with the nipple shield* (our emphasis). She has been on the bottle now for 11 weeks. Is it possible to get her back to the breast and what is the success rate using a nipple shield because I really miss that feeling of having her close to me?

This mother wants to get back on the nipple shield, which caused the decrease in her milk supply in the first place! Another mother's baby did gain well but there were other issues with nipple shields. (Capitals are in the original email.)

> My 10-week-old daughter is still on the nipple shield, and I have tried EVERYTHING to wean her off. I had a HORRIBLE experience with all the consultants at Xxxxxx Hospital. She had trouble latching on at birth, but instead of working with me, I think I got 5 minutes before they threw the shield at me. Being drained and emotional, I took it not having anybody there telling me anything else. I'm grateful she's getting my milk, gaining weight, and healthy. However, I'm getting to the point where I'm nervous about joining a mom's group or breastfeeding ANYWHERE in public due to it being super awkward to feed with the shield. I'm starting to think our whole breastfeeding experience is going to be on the shield, which frustrates me. I just want to exhaust all my options, and make sure that there's nothing else wrong (tongue-tie, etc.) before I commit to keep going with the shield. Thank you!!

Health professionals recommend nipple shields without regard to the long-term consequences. They are sometimes used when babies initially refuse the breast. However, these same babies easily latch on when the milk flow increases on day 3 or 4. Latching on well depends on the mother producing an abundant milk supply. Artificial nipples (nipple shields) can impede the development of an abundant supply.

## Hospital Staff Has Less Experience with Hands-On Help

Another problem is that the more hospital staff use nipple shields, the less proficient they become in helping mothers latch on babies. Nipple-shields are attractive because they *seem to work* immediately. To be provocative, when hospital staff give mothers nipple shields soon after birth, staff gets to pass the problem on to someone else once the mother and baby are discharged from hospital. Frequently no-one even perceives there is a problem, so the mother is not directed to the help she needs. It can be weeks before we see babies in our clinic, and by then, it's much more difficult to help the mother latch the baby on directly to the breast.

## Misdiagnosis of Flat Nipples

Health professionals also use nipple shields for mothers with "flat nipples." One mother wrote this.

> I have a 12-week-old baby girl. I breastfed for the first week after her birth with a nipple shield because I have very flat, small nipples.

We saw another mother at the clinic who received nipple shields while she was on the delivery table. This mother did not have flat nipples; they were normal, but they looked flat when the mother was lying down, and her breasts were engorged with IV fluids. Too many mothers are given nipple shields for the same specious reasoning, before they have even tried getting the baby on the breast. Mothers sometimes get misdiagnosed with flat nipples because:

- The mother received intravenous fluids during labor, which caused edema of the nipples and areolas.
- The hospital staff has not been trained to accurately diagnose what normal nipples look like. Even so called "inverted nipples" do not necessarily prevent the baby latching on.

## A Tool for Teaching the Baby to Breastfeed?

Some people believe that nipple shields teach babies, especially preterm babies, how to breastfeed. This is pure fantasy! The mind boggles! Babies on a nipple shield are not latched on at all, so how can this teach them to breastfeed? The question is, if a nipple shield is just like breastfeeding, why will a baby seemingly "take the breast" with a nipple shield and not take the breast directly? Instead of the baby latching on to the soft, supple, pliable breast, which is an active process, they latch on to a nipple shield, which is neither soft, supple, nor pliable, and is essentially pushed into the baby's mouth. The nipple shield turns the breast into a bottle. It's no more complicated than that. With a nipple shield in their mouths, babies use their tongues and cheek muscles just as they do with a bottle or pacifier, *not* the way they would when breastfeeding.

Some lactation consultants argue that nipple shields give new mothers confidence and hope. How this actually works is beyond us. Nipple shields make mothers, and their helpers believe that their breastfeeding problems have been solved. To repeat, a baby on a nipple shield is not latched on at all, and the nipple shield certainly does not correct a tongue-tie.

## Safety and Efficacy of Their Use

The epidemic of nipple-shield use has happened without any evidence supporting it. This review from *Breastfeeding Medicine* summarizes research up to 2010 (McKechnie & Eglash, 2010). The authors concluded that nipple shields were neither safe nor effective.

> Introducing nipple shields in the first postpartum week may seem like an easy fix for a frustrated family, but such an intervention may preclude a thorough evaluation of the mother/infant dyad to determine why breastfeeding has been problematic and may cause more problems, such as lack of effective milk transfer, sore nipples, and loss of milk supply. The pervasive use of nipple shields as an intervention in the very early course of breastfeeding can relay a false message of breastfeeding success and safety to mothers. Widespread retail access to nipple shields might also signal to mothers that nipple shield use is a norm that warrants little concern. In clinical medicine, it is generally accepted that one must prove the safety and usefulness of an intervention before one can generally recommend it. Nipple shield use has never been proved safe or effective (McKechnie & Eglash, 2010) (p. 613).

Of course, some have managed to feed their babies up to age 6 months, or even longer, with a nipple shield. We argue that they have managed *despite*, not because of, the nipple shield. Why? Because their milk supply and flow were still abundant. Most mothers cannot continue with nipple shields and as a result, either stop breastfeeding or decide to pump exclusively.

## What Could Be Done Instead?

Based on combined 55 years of helping mothers, we believe that anything that can be done with a nipple shield is better without one. If a baby can latch on to a nipple shield, for example, the baby should be able to latch on to the breast. Here an example of how to coax a reluctant baby to the breast.

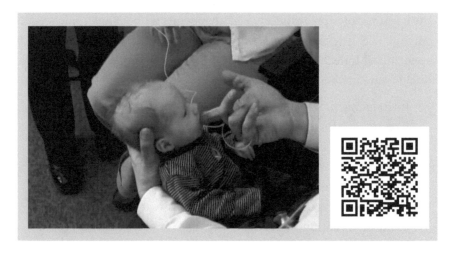

Unfortunately, patience is necessary to solve some breastfeeding problems: both from mothers and their helpers. If need be, we can wait a few days for babies to latch on while feeding the baby expressed milk by cup, spoon, or if necessary, slow-flow bottle.

## Conclusions

In our experience, nipple shields lower milk supply because babies are not latched on to the breast. They are also difficult to stop using once babies get used to their feel and flow. Many practitioners use nipple shields to quickly "solve" breastfeeding problems, but they often create more problems than they solve. Therefore, we do not recommend using nipple shields.

# MILK SUPPLY

# CHAPTER 14

# Is the Baby Getting Enough to Eat? Assessing Infant Weight Gain

Physicians consider babies' weight gain as the ideal way of knowing whether babies are getting enough to eat. It's the first commandment of infant feeding. Physicians' training emphasizes it. Rules like, "the baby needs to gain 30 grams (1 ounce) a day in the first few months after birth" have been drilled into their heads from the first day they worked with young babies. Adequate weight gain means that babies double their birthweight by 4 months and triple it by a year.

Mothers often tell us that the doctor is concerned because the baby gained, for example, only 26 grams in a day rather than 30. Given the frequent mistakes made weighing babies, this is pseudoscience at its worst. A baby steadily gaining 4 grams a day less than the "ideal" 30 g/day will be fine. They may be a bit thin, but as long as the baby continues to grow, there is no need to worry. Yet parents we meet are frequently told that lower weight gain causes brain damage! Not surprisingly, they are often scared to death. We will say this unequivocally; steadily growing babies will *not* be brain damaged even if their rate of growth is slower than what is considered "ideal."

## What Happens When Doctors Are Concerned?

Doctors are quick to tell mothers whose babies have slow weight gain to use bottles of formula. Few doctors try to help the breastfeeding to go better.

"Give the baby a bottle after each breastfeed" is the common suggestion. Unfortunately, bottles usually lead to deterioration of the breastfeeding relationship and frequently, to complete breast refusal. Basically, bottles do not improve the way a baby latches on. If anything, artificial nipples worsen latch, even when the bottle contains breastmilk. Some babies will take both breast and bottle, but we insist that even if the baby does, using bottles steadily decreases how much milk they take from the breast.

Another absurd routine is when an exclusively breastfeeding baby is not gaining weight, so the physician, public-health nurse, or lactation consultant urges the mother to use an exhausting regimen. Feed the baby on the breast for X minutes on each side, pump her breasts, and feed the expressed milk (or formula if "enough" is not expressed) by bottle. Once the baby is gaining weight well, the mother is told she can now feed the baby just on the breast, which does not work, because the initial problem causing slow weight gain was not addressed.

Here is another approach that some doctors recommend for slow weight gain, from a mother's email.

Dr says baby is not gaining fast enough & that I will need to supplement with formula if baby has not gained enough by the next few appointments (he wants me to go in for a weekly weight check).

According to the mother's email, the doctor has suggested nothing more than that. This is not a rare approach in dealing with slow weight gain for some doctors. See the mother and baby every week until the mother is worn down and convinced the baby needs to be supplemented. Again, everything is based on the scale with no practical help. The doctor is, I (JN) am guessing now, pleased with him/herself because s/he is giving the mother and baby every chance, but knows what will happen after a few weeks at the most. After all, if nothing changes in how the baby is being fed, why will the baby start to gain enough weight?

## What Healthcare Providers Should Do Instead

We recommend that health professionals include other metrics, and not just weight gain, to determine if babies are eating enough. Using weight alone can lead to errors. To begin with, healthcare providers should watch babies at the breast to determine whether they are drinking well at the breast.

Unfortunately, most health professionals have never learned, and do not know how to assess babies at the breast. Most are completely oblivious that such a thing is possible. Indeed, most do not know that they need more information than the baby's weight. Many, in fact the vast majority, assume that if babies have breasts in their mouths and are making sucking motions, that they are receiving milk. This is simply *not* true. A baby may be latched on and making sucking movements but getting very little milk from the breast. Without knowing how to assess whether babies are drinking at the breast, health professionals will continue to give mothers poor advice that leads to breastfeeding failure. Poor advice also comes from family, friends, and even strangers, but health professionals are the ones who should know how to help. If they don't, they need to find someone who does or resolve to learn about breastfeeding themselves.

### Our Approach

After assessing babies at the breast, we help the mother improve the latch. We teach her how to know when her baby *drinks* at the breast and how to use breast compressions to increase the flow of milk to the baby. When breast compressions no longer increase flow, the mother should offer the baby her other breast, and then possibly offer the first breast again. We then ask the mother to follow-up within a few days to a week, depending on how well our approach seemed to work. We do not hesitate to use domperidone, which may be part of the treatment plan, but not the only treatment. This is a quick summary of how we deal with the baby not getting enough from the breast. We provide more detail throughout this book.

## Growth Curves

Oh, the growth chart! They are useful tools *if used properly*, but it is amazing how they can be misused. Here is an email from the father of a baby.

> We have a 4½-month-old baby. He weighs 13.1 lbs (5.95 kg), 27" (69 cm) long. He is a very healthy and happy baby. The doctor has said that the baby is underweight, and he is at the 35% percentile in weight compared to other babies. My wife wants to stop breastfeeding and give him formula because she wants the baby to gain weight.

Interestingly, there is no 35th percentile line so this "scientific" number is a bit of a guess. I (JN) write back saying that you cannot look at just one percentile and that if the baby was always on the 35th percentile, this is normal, but if the baby's weight is slipping downward, this could be an issue. In his second email, the father said,

> To answer your question, the baby went from being in the 25% percentile at the end of the 3rd month to being in the 35% at 4½ months.

And guess what? The mother did stop breastfeeding. This is mind boggling. Does this doctor think that all babies should be at the 50th percentile or higher? By definition, this is impossible and not how growth charts work. Someone, someone *normal,* has to be on the 3rd percentile, or 5th percentile, or 20th percentile. If you believe this is a one-off case, you are mistaken. This sort of doctor advice is far from rare. Reflect on this quotation.

> Science is rooted in creative interpretation ... Theories are built upon the interpretation of numbers, and interpreters are often trapped by their own rhetoric ... and fail to discern the prejudice that leads them to one interpretation among many consistent with their numbers. —Stephen Jay Gould (1996), *The Mismeasure of Man*

We believe that this doctor was so convinced that babies need to be at the 50th percentile or higher that he ignored the evidence of a thriving baby who was right in front of him.

## When the Growth Curve Says Everything is Fine, and It Is Not

Here is another example of a growth-curve mistake. This case, several years ago, turned on a light for us. We learned that babies can still be hungry, even if they are growing well. The baby was breastfeeding exclusively, and on observation, drinking well at the breast. The baby's weight gain was "perfect" in grams/day, and the growth curve was spot-on perfect. Yet, he was crying constantly. We saw the baby twice at around 2 months. We tried various techniques, including improving the latch, using breast compressions and so on, without a change. The evening before the third visit, the mother, exhausted by the baby's almost constant crying, gave him a bottle of formula and the baby calmed down. We admit, we were baffled. The next day, at the scheduled follow-up appointment, we tried using the lactation aid at the breast to supplement with formula. The baby fed well and came off the breast calm for the very first time in his life. He just wanted more milk, no matter how well he was gaining. If supplementation is necessary, as it was in this case to help us understand what was going on, the supplement should be given by a lactation aid at the breast, as this results in continued breastfeeding. It is likely also that this baby and mother would have benefited from the mother taking domperidone.

## Scales and Weighing Can Lead to Misinterpretation

We always weigh babies at our clinic, but we do so *only* as a check on our observations of the baby at the breast. If something does not fit, we make clinical decisions based on the mother's feeding history and our observations of *how the baby drinks at the breast*. Of course, even observing the baby at the breast is not always perfect. We frequently encounter this situation.

> I had to feed the baby in the car just before we arrived at the clinic. S/he was screaming and I just could not hold her off.

The following case study shows how basing everything on the weight leads to misunderstanding.

> The baby is 1 month old. I (AP) suggested the mother had had a decrease in her milk flow.

Late onset decreasing milk flow typically, in our practice, presents at 3 to 4 months of age. However, we have seen babies presenting at 1 month, or even 3 weeks of age, with this problem. I (JN) used to be puzzled by mothers asking, "Everything was fine, the baby was happy and gaining well, but then, around 3 weeks of age, he became fussy and even refused to latch on." There seems to be such a thing as "early onset, late onset decreasing milk supply and flow."

The mother went to see her pediatrician who weighed the baby. The baby gained 240 g in the past week. The pediatrician convinced the mother that I, the lactation consultant, was wrong, that the baby indeed had reflux and the mother had too much milk. That was the reason why the baby was pulling off the breast and crying.

"Too much milk"? Another myth!

The pediatrician referred the mother to the hospital for an ultrasound to confirm the reflux. Today the mother went to see the pediatrician to discuss the results of the ultrasound. The baby was weighed and in the past two days was down 100g.

Incidentally, an ultrasound does not confirm reflux, since, when doing an ultrasound babies lie on their backs, they frequently show "reflux" but in fact, are normal. Even if babies' "beds" are perpendicular, pushing on their abdomen with the ultrasound probe shows "reflux."

Now the pediatrician panicked and according to the mother: "did blood work to make sure my baby was healthy."

What blood work makes sure the baby is healthy? Whatever happened to examining the baby?

Then the pediatrician instructed the mother to weigh her before and after feedings and to "only express my milk and feed her by bottle to find out whether my baby has difficulty getting the milk from the breast even though the milk is there" (*Babies suck milk out of the breast?*). "Or whether she requires supplementation because the milk is not there."

Remember that babies often get more from the breast than most mothers can pump. The poor baby in this case gets an *unnecessary ultrasound, goes through the pain of blood work,* and his mother is now scared to death that the baby is truly sick. All of this could have been avoided if they had watched the baby at the breast.

Here's another example of how weighing can provide misinformation. A postpartum doula shared this story.

> …how weighing can make things seem good (*or in other situations, can make things seem bad*). So, on for first day after birth the baby was weighed, 2880 g (6lb 5oz). On the second day of life, today, the baby was weighed on the same scale and the weight was 2960 g (6lb 8oz). The nurses were impressed. But they should not have been. I was present both times and the first day the baby was weighed naked. On the second day, the baby was weighed with her diaper on plus a cloth diaper spread on the scale. I tried to explain but they said: "Don't worry, this is very good."

It is incredible that given the various problems with weighing that this postpartum unit failed to follow a standard weighing approach.

## Yet Another Example of the Tyranny of the Scale

This email comes in when the baby is 7 days old. The mother is still supplementing.

> Within 36 hours of his birth, he had lost 9% of his weight, a fact which threw the nurses on the labour ward into a *panicked flurry of activity* (our emphasis). Within minutes of having weighed him, I was hooked up to a breast pump, and being shown how to use the feeding tubes and syringe to supplement my baby with formula.

Our comment: Syringe for an improvised lactation aid? Why? Answer: So milk can be pushed into the baby's mouth in this "dire emergency." By email, I (JN) suggested the mother follow the *Protocol to Manage Breastmilk Intake* (Newman, 2021) and use the video clips to help her use the Protocol. We received this email 2 weeks later.

Thank you once again for your help and advice. We have been following the steps in the *Protocol to Manage Breastmilk Intake* and have had wonderful success! We are no longer supplementing, and our baby boy is gaining plenty of weight.

### Some Questions

- ◊ Is it likely that a mother who has enough milk at 3 weeks, despite a terrible start, does not have enough colostrum?

- ◊ Would the mother have benefited from *good* help breastfeeding in the hospital?

- ◊ What could the hospital staff have done instead of "panicked flurry of activity"?

- ◊ What might explain the weight loss even if the baby truly lost 9% of the birthweight?

- ◊ What would have happened to most mothers?

Watch this video. The baby in this video is 10% below birthweight. Is the baby drinking well? Yes. Does the baby need supplementation as the hospital nurse recommends? No.

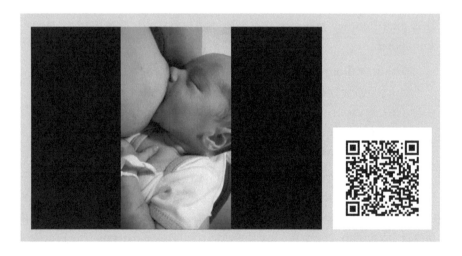

This baby latched (photos below) on well after birth but was then given bottles for a 10% weight loss. After that, he no longer latched on. His mother had a caesarean section for meconium after 14 hours of labor. The baby has obvious swelling of the face and the rest of his body (see photo on the left). The baby also had an obvious tongue-tie, but this was ignored. We can also ask why is this baby in an incubator instead of skin to skin with his mother?

We saw the baby because he was not latching on. He was being fed breastmilk exclusively and was gaining weight well. The 2nd photo on the right is at our clinic at 2 weeks of age. He is no longer swollen and is calm and alert.

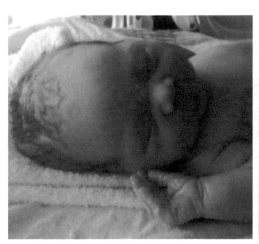 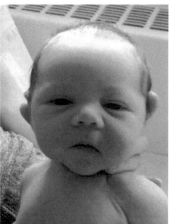

## Exclusively Breastfed Babies Can Grow and Thrive

Some doctors truly believe that exclusive breastfeeding rarely works, and that babies are in constant danger of starvation. Yes, we need to be vigilant and make sure breastfeeding gets off to a good start, but it does work. We would like to show you some babies from our practice. The below shows a 6-month-old baby who has been *exclusively breastfed* since birth, *except* for a few bottles of formula (mother could not remember how many) in the hospital because of a 10% weight loss.

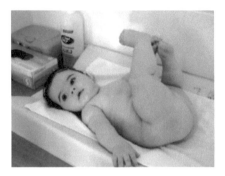

Here's another baby. He is a 5-month-old who was exclusively breastfed once he left hospital. Baby was given formula by bottle because he was not latching on. (What happened to expressing the mother's milk?)

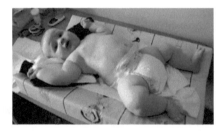

This following photo shows a 6-month-old baby, exclusively breastfeeding except for a few bottles of formula in hospital for 10% weight loss. Birthweight was 3.81 kg (8lb 6oz). Weight at the time of the photo 8.94 kg (19lb 11oz). Does this require an explanation?

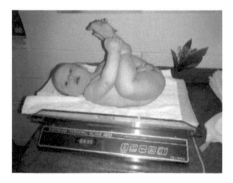

We hope you can see that with good support and proper assessment, most babies grow and thrive on exclusive breastfeeding alone.

## Managing Slow Weight Gain

The baby in this video was brought to our clinic for slow weight gain. After our recommended adjustments, the baby was drinking well enough. We decided not to do anything more but asked the mother to return in 2 days. However, the baby *did not gain any weight at all* from the first to the second visit, only 2 days later, but he also did not lose weight, he was the same.

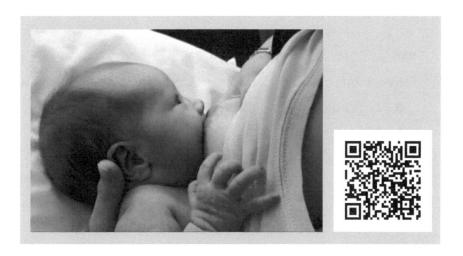

Remember, weighing after 2 days is not especially useful, even on the same scale. The baby may have had a large bowel movement, or spat up, or urinated (or all three). What really counts is that the baby *drank much better* than at the second visit than he did the first (i.e., he showed longer pauses and had a better response to breast compressions). We decided to see him again in another week.

A week after the second visit, the baby drank very well, with virtually no need for the mother to do breast compressions. For those who like weights, the baby gained 250 grams (a little more than 1/2 pound) in the week. With email follow-up, the mother and baby were able to breastfeed exclusively to 6 months or so, with good weight gain. At about 6 months, the baby started eating food, after which, we had no more communication.

It helped that we saw the baby at 2 weeks of age. Unfortunately, too many of our referrals, including those for slow weight gain, sore nipples, babies not latching on, come much later. We often don't see babies who are not gaining well until 7, 8, or even 12 weeks after birth. By then, they are almost universally receiving bottles. The bottles may contain expressed milk, but bottles teach babies a latch that is inappropriate for breastfeeding. Thus, breastfeeding problems are frequently difficult to turn around. The problem self-perpetuates. If the baby takes the breast with a poor latch, milk supply and flow will decrease. Early intervention makes a huge difference.

## A Strange Case

Here is another case that taught us a lot. Below are the baby's weights.

- Birthweight: 3.555 kg (7lb 14oz)
- Day 3: 3.5 kg (7lb 11.5oz)
- Day 4: 3.6 kg (7lb 15oz)
- Day 8: 3.79 kg (8lb 5.7oz)
- Day 23: 4.78 kg (10lb 8oz)

Now watch the video.

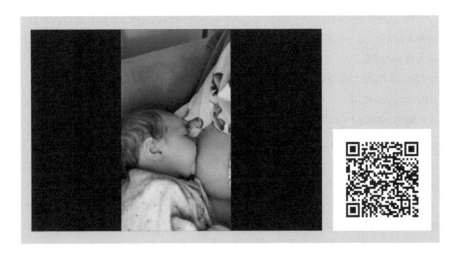

First of all, the baby is not latched on well. The latch is symmetrical, and the baby does not have a lot of breast in his mouth. More importantly, though, he has *some* sucks with short pauses, and as a result, we are not confident that the weights are accurate. It is difficult to believe that a baby with this kind of latch, who is drinking so little, though there were some pausing type sucks, could gain almost a kilogram (2.2 pounds) in 15 days. Something is surely wrong here and does not make sense. Indeed, the midwife contacted us because the baby was going to the breast *at least* 16 times a day.

What happened? The baby continued to gain weight well while exclusively breastfeeding. I (JN) was very surprised, though I guess I should not have been. I (AP) correctly stated that the baby would gain weight well. The baby was on the breast virtually 24 hours a day, and maybe that's what did it. However, with a better latch, I am sure the baby could have breastfed less frequently, and things would have been easier for both mother and baby.

## Can a Baby Gain Too Much?

With all the concern about childhood obesity, some mothers (and doctors) worry that breastfed babies will get fat. There's good news here. While you can overfeed a bottle-fed baby, you cannot overfeed an exclusively breastfeeding one. Yet people worry. Here is an email from a breastfeeding mother.

> I saw my baby's pediatrician and he said that she is way too big for her age (5 months). That I should stop breastfeeding overnight and give her water instead, to start solid food now so she breastfeeds less and to start iron liquid supplement without having any blood test done prior to it. Is there an issue or consequences in the long term if my baby girl is "obese" now? Is it dangerous for her to be that big with my milk?

Once again, the scale is everything, the only thing that matters, and once again, the pediatrician does not understand breastfeeding babies. How is this mother going to stop breastfeeding at night? By giving the baby water? The baby does not want water. The baby wants breastfeeding, especially, the *relationship* of breastfeeding, yes even at 5 months of age. It is also unlikely that giving the baby solids at 5 months will decrease the baby's frequency of breastfeeding. This pediatrician does not understand that babies do not breastfeed *only* for food. Giving the baby water at night will lead to an inconsolable crying baby.

Here is another case report of an "overweight" baby. We agree that a case report does not *prove* much. Nevertheless, it suggests that "overweight babies" tend to slim down as they get older. The mother of the baby in photos attached wrote:

> He was born 9lbs 8oz (4.32 kg) at a little over 37 weeks gestation (No gestational diabetes) and reached 20lbs (9.1kg) by the time he was 10 weeks old! Now at 2 he is only 30lbs (13.6 kg). I'm very fortunate that my pediatrician took it all in stride and never recommended changing our feeding patterns!

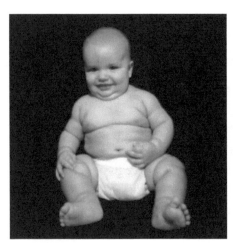 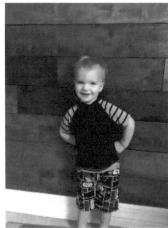

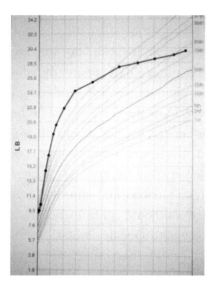

This is the email from a mother of an 8-week-old baby.

> My baby's pediatrician told me that my 8-week-old baby is gaining too much weight. My 8-week-old is on the 98th centile for height and weight and that she is becoming a fat baby. I breastfeed on demand. My pediatrician advised me I need to space out the feeds. My baby will cry until she is fed.

This pediatrician understands neither breastfeeding nor growth charts, which is surprising as pediatricians spend a lot of time learning to interpret growth charts. Somebody has got to be on the 98th percentile. We've always said that though some exclusively breastfed babies grow very quickly on breastfeeding alone, sometimes to the point where people worry, they tend to slim down as they get older.

I remember one case at the Hospital for Sick Children (Toronto) when I (JN) was working in the emergency department. A 7-month-old baby arrived with mild respiratory distress. She weighed 22.7 kg (50 lb). The respiratory distress was not a big deal, but the mother was threatened with child protection services if she did not stop breastfeeding the baby so frequently (10 or 12 times a day, apparently, which is not really *that* frequent). The mother did not listen and kept doing what she had always done. Three years later, I saw the child at a La Leche League conference. The child was tall for her age, but not abnormally so, and was of average weight for her height. The lesson from this case is not everyone fits into the same box. People vary. Indeed, trying to squeeze everyone into the same box makes parents anxious, and some will even stop breastfeeding. In short, breastfed babies should control when and how much they eat. Incidentally, but maybe not so incidentally, I am still shocked years later at how this mother and child were treated.

## Is Serum Sodium a Good Measure Baby's Intake?

Some pediatricians like to measure babies' serum sodium to determine whether they are getting enough from the breast. We could find no articles in English that support this. Laing and Wong (2002) note that babies with severe dehydration due to insufficient intake have elevated sodium levels. High, but normal levels of sodium were more common in formula-fed infants, apparently, but are sodium levels a test for dehydration? If babies are significantly dehydrated, there are prominent physical signs and historical information, which are much better than serum sodium. Serum sodium can help us decide how to manage intravenous rehydration, but not in making the diagnosis.

Let us think about this a bit. Do we even know what the *normal* serum sodium levels are in an exclusively breastfed baby at 3 or 4 days of life? Maybe someone has studied that, but we could not find such a study. The serum sodium does not help if we do not observe the baby at the breast.

Exclusively breastfed babies *normally* receive smaller amounts of milk compared to artificially fed babies. So, how can we expect breastfed babies' serum sodium to be the same as formula-fed babies who drink significantly larger amounts? Given the relative volumes, the serum sodium is likely higher in the exclusively breastfed baby. Does that mean that they are not getting enough volume? (Note: the exclusively breastfed baby is the model of normal, not the formula-fed baby). We really do not know what the normal serum sodium in the exclusively breastfed baby between day 3 of life and day 10, say, but if the baby is drinking well and looking and acting like a healthy newborn, why search for problems that don't exist?

Another monkey wrench to consider when interpreting sodium levels: the intravenous fluids the mother (and the baby) received during labor. High volume of fluid decreases the baby's serum sodium. Babies who received a lot of fluids will have a lower serum sodium, but does that mean that they are getting enough to eat? Impossible to say without observing the baby at the breast.

What we don't understand is why people propose all these methods of measuring babies' intake at the breast, when almost always, watching babies at the breast (plus some history) tells us all we need to know.

## Conclusion

Physicians consider weight gain a key indicator of babies' well-being. If babies' weights falter, they are often quick to recommend formula. We believe that weight is also an important marker and should be used to confirm what we see when we watch as the mother breastfeeds, but that weight measurement can be prone to error and should not be the sole metric. Assessment should include watching babies at the breast to see if they are latched on and drinking well. We teach mothers to use breast compressions and offer the second breast (and then back to the first). If necessary, we will also prescribe domperidone.

# CHAPTER 15

# Late Onset Decreasing Milk Supply and Flow

We first recognized this as a "syndrome" around 2013. Since then, we see two or three mothers every day who fit the picture. This syndrome presents in various ways and is usually misdiagnosed as reflux, colic, or an allergy to something in the mother's milk, usually cows' milk protein. We believe none of these diagnoses is correct if babies are exclusively breastfed from birth, as they often are, because this "syndrome" is characteristic of mothers who start off with an abundant milk supply.

Late onset decreased milk supply and flow does not *necessarily* mean "not enough milk," a notion that is often difficult for the mother to accept as she often believed she had an "overabundance of milk." In fact, what many consider an overabundance is nothing of the kind, but rather a baby who cannot handle a rapid flow of milk because the baby's latch is not as good as it could be. This notion of the milk supply being overabundant can be explained by a good milk supply when the baby's latch is not as good as it could be. Indeed, when the mother's milk is abundant, often the baby does not have to latch on well to get enough milk to grow well, at least at first. If the baby's latch is not as good as it could be, the mother's milk supply could easily decrease and the symptoms of late onset decreasing milk supply and flow become evident. Evident to us, but not to most doctors.

Indeed, the mother's milk supply may still be reasonably good, and the baby often continues to gain weight fairly well, at least if diagnosis and treatment is not too long delayed. The difference is that the baby has been used to a faster flow and is now not happy with a slower flow. This situation could be likened to breastfeeding babies who had bottles of breastmilk.

They got used to the regular, steady flow of the bottle. Mothers report that their babies started to "not to like the breast." Eventually, with no intervention, babies will not get enough from the breast.

The following videos show a 3-month-old baby during different parts of the same feeding session. The mother and baby were doing very well for the first weeks, but then the baby stopped being calm at the breast. The mother had had a large milk supply (from history) and the flow of milk to the baby was good at first. In the videos, the baby's latch looks fairly good (in the first video, except that the lower lip is sucked in a bit, suggesting, we think, that the baby had a tongue-tie, which she did.) A tongue-tie results in a poor latch. So, even though the mother started off with no problems, breastfeeding deteriorated, so that by the time of these videos at 3 months of age, after a short period of decent drinking (video 1), the baby fusses and pulls at the breast when the flow of milk slows (Video 3).

**Video 1**

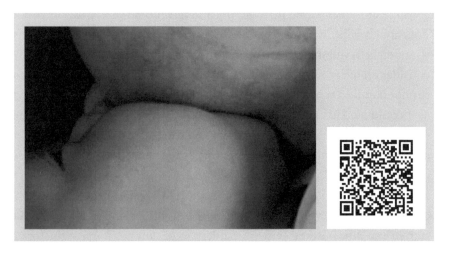

The baby is drinking relatively well in Video 2. There are pauses as the baby opens to the widest point, but we would like to see *longer* pauses. Note the lower lip is sucked in and not splayed out the way it normally should be.

**Video 2**

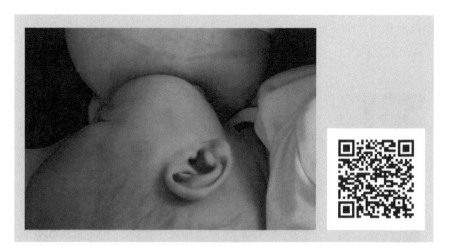

Video 2 shows somewhat less drinking than Video 1. We asked the mother to start breast compressions to keep up the flow of milk. The compressions help somewhat, but the baby is already pulling a little at the breast.

**Video 3**

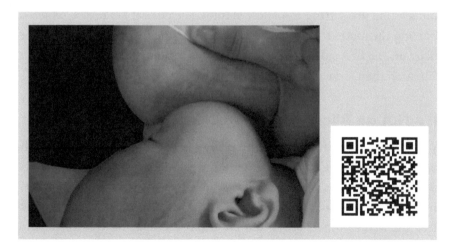

In Video 3, breast compressions are still working somewhat. The lactation consultant says that when the baby asks for more, the mother should start the compressions. To be accurate, the baby does not really "ask for the milk," obviously. Rather, the baby was fussing in response to the milk's slower flow. The clicking may be the baby releasing the breast.

**Video 4**

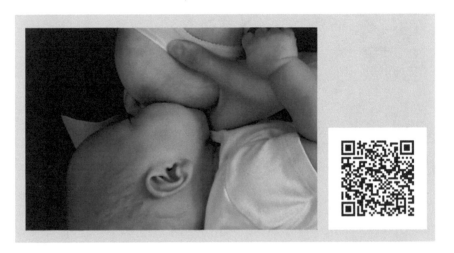

In Video 4, compressions are working less and less and the effect on the drinking is less and less. The baby is squirming at the breast and is still hungry, but not getting good flow of milk. She pulls at the breast, which is hurting the mother. Time to switch sides. Telling the mother to keep the baby on the first side for 10 or 20 minutes makes no more sense in this situation than it does for any mother/baby pair.

## It's Not an Allergy

We believe that what many call an allergy is late onset decreasing supply and flow. Babies are fussy because they are not getting good flow of milk at the breast. Babies' symptoms are not due to an allergen in the mothers' milk (Medical dictum: "never say never"). Most had been exclusively breastfeeding. Many of their babies did not even receive a bottle of formula in the hospital, which is rather unusual in Southern Ontario. An allergy to something in the milk seems unlikely.

Cows' milk is the most common allergen that mothers have been asked to remove from their diet, followed by soy, then a whole range of other foods. Some breastfeeding mothers are close to a diet of water only, yet their babies usually do not improve. If following a strict diet does not improve the baby's symptoms, "special formula" is the next recommendation by the pediatrician, and the baby gets better. Everyone is convinced, even the parents. Why does the baby get better? Not because the formula is "hypo-allergenic," but because the baby now gets steady flow of milk and a *full feeding*. Following that logic, babies would improve on ordinary formula. Here is a what happened to one mother whose baby was diagnosed with allergy to breastmilk because the baby was having blood in the bowel movements.

> My baby had blood in stool a few months ago. The physician suspect-ed milk-protein allergy and had me eliminate dairy from my diet. You wrote me back that it was more likely late onset decreased milk supply. I was started on domperidone 90 mg daily. My milk supply dropped again, so the dose of domperidone was increased to 120 mg (12 pills) daily and we saw the lactation consultant. She diagnosed tongue-tie causing shallow latch. The tongue-tie was released by a pediatrician one month later.

Note: It took a month to release the tongue-tie?

> At this point things were now perfect. I started dairy products again three weeks ago. I decreased the dose of domperidone from 120 mg/day to 40 mg daily by 10 mg every 3 days.

*Our comment: this is much too rapidly. We recommend decreasing the dose by 10 mg a week, so that if the mother was taking 120 mg, she would take 110 mg for a week, then 100 mg for a week and so on.*

> Milk supply dropped. Two days later, blood in stool again and off and on for 3 days now. I upped my domperidone to 90 mg daily again. My baby had milk proteins for 3 weeks and no blood. Is it safe to assume it's not an allergy causing bloody stool?

*I (JN) never thought it was an allergy to something in the milk.*

## Causes of Late Onset Decreasing Milk Supply and Flow

Late onset decreasing milk supply and flow seems to occur most frequently in mothers who started out with an abundant milk supply, but for some reason, the supply (and flow) decreased. Babies may continue to gain weight well, though if the situation is not fixed, eventually the weight gain will slow. The key is *how babies react to the decreased flow*, even if they continue to gain weight well. If they are fussy at the breast, on a "nursing strike" (baby refusing to latch on even if hungry), or sucking their fingers much of the time, then things are definitely not okay. Interestingly, these babies *tend* to breastfeed best at night.

### Bad Advice Can Lower Supply

If mothers have abundant supplies and babies do not latch on well, babies will be unable to handle the rapid flow of milk and may choke and sputter. Many lactation consultants diagnose "oversupply." Instead of dealing with the problem, which is usually the baby's less than ideal latch, many physicians and lactation consultants recommend feeding the baby on only one breast at each feeding to slow the flow of milk by decreasing supply. Well, this works as far as decreasing the supply, and it often works *too well*, because the mother's milk supply and the flow of milk decrease—exactly the problem we are discussing here.

### One-Sided Feeding

This notion arises from the fact that fat content in milk increases as the baby *drinks* longer at the breast, so doctors (and lactation consultants) tell mothers to feed on only one breast at a feeding, sometimes even several times on the same breast (see below). The secret is this: *if babies are not drinking at the breast, they are not getting high-fat milk no matter how long they suck on the breast.*

Mothers are frequently surprised and resist believing what has happened. They may say, "I have always had a lot of milk," or "I can pump 180 ml (6 oz) any time I want," or "he's gaining lots of weight." Mothers' objections do not change the problem related to one-sided feeding. If babies have good weight gain without other problems, then one-sided feeding is not a problem but should not be the 11th commandment. Mothers should feed on the first side until the baby is not drinking any longer, and the baby should then be offered the other breast. Nevertheless, the mother should routinely offer the second breast.

We hear far too often that babies will not take the second breast if they are offered it. This occurs, usually, because the mother keeps the baby on the first breast until the baby is fast asleep. The mother should offer the second breast when the baby is no longer drinking not when he has fallen into deep sleep. If offered the breast when relatively awake and not drinking, babies may or may not take the second breast, depending on whether they are still hungry.

### Block Feeding

Some mothers are being counseled to "block feed," meaning that they feed the baby several times in a row on the same breast without offering the other breast. After a "set" number of feedings on one side, the mother can start offering the other breast. How the "set number of times" is determined is beyond us. However, one thing is for sure, the milk supply and flow of milk to the baby will decrease, often rapidly.

Babies' choking at the breast is a sign that the baby is not well latched on and as a result cannot handle the rapid flow. Not because there is too much milk! With a good latch, babies can handle a rapid flow of milk. Feeding one breast at a feeding or block feeding will decrease milk supply and flow, so choking becomes less frequent, but other problems arise, specifically, late onset decreased milk supply and flow, and often, late onset nipple soreness.

### Artificial Nipples

Bottles, pacifiers, and nipple shields can significantly decrease milk supply and flow of milk when used routinely, even if it is breastmilk in the bottle. This problem occurs where mothers do not have adequate maternity leave and need to return to work before their babies can drink from a cup (the truth is that even premature babies can drink from a cup but unfortunately many daycare workers freak out at the idea of cup feeding even 1 year old babies).

Even when mothers have decent maternity leave, when fathers, partners, or others feed the baby, milk supply decreases. Some mothers attending our breastfeeding clinic have had the father feeding the baby bottles of expressed milk during the night, sometimes all night, while the mother, awake at the same time, expresses her milk. The point of this is beyond us though I know why this happens. However, the mother's partner can bond with babies in so many ways besides by feeding the baby. Babies have other needs besides feedings. And the father can feed the baby when the baby is eating food after 6 months of age.

### Medications

Some medications decrease the milk supply and flow. These include birth control pills and intrauterine devices with progesterone. The fact that not all mothers seem to have a decrease does not nullify the observation.

Clomiphene and letrozole used in fertility treatments also decrease the milk supply significantly. Some drugs such as bromocriptine and cabergoline apparently can decrease the milk supply drastically, or even shut it off completely. These drugs are apparently commonly used in some eastern European countries for the treatment of postpartum engorgement, a completely inappropriate and senseless use for these conditions, which should be treated with improving the baby's latch.

Antihistamines, especially the older ones like diphenhydramine (Benadryl), as well as possibly pseudoephedrine, can also decrease milk supply, even when taken only once. Newer antihistamines *may* not cause a decrease with emphasis on "may." There are other treatments for allergies other than antihistamines. For self-limited allergies, such as poison ivy, prednisone in low doses (say, 5 mg three times a day or 2 with slow tapering over a week or so) seems to work well and does not decrease the milk supply, while giving the mother effective relief.

### Sleep Training

Sleep training is used to "help" babies sleep through the night. But it often results in decreasing milk supply and flow. For many babies, night feedings are when they get most of their milk intake. Eliminating or significantly decreasing night feedings may result in late onset decreasing milk flow. Indeed, with late onset decreasing milk supply, it is often the night feedings that keep the baby gaining weight well. Cutting down or eliminating night feedings will often result in much more rapid decrease in milk supply and flow.

## Symptoms of Late Onset Decreasing Milk Supply and Flow

Late onset decreasing milk supply and flow is a *progressive* problem. Symptoms often start out subtly and worsen progressively without early intervention. By the time babies are 3 months of age, they may completely refuse the breast during the day, though they may still take the breast at night.

### Shorter Evening Feedings

Mothers may interpret shorter evening feedings as the baby becoming more efficient at breastfeeding, filling up more quickly than when they were younger. The notion of babies becoming more efficient at the breast is puzzling. It seems that more efficient babies means that babies pull milk out of the breast better at 3 months, rather than 3 weeks, except that babies don't pull milk out of the breast. Mothers may think this is a good thing that the feedings are shorter, but often this change is the beginning of an increase in symptoms that become progressively more worrisome.

### Decreased Frequency of Bowel Movements

Another possible symptom is an early decrease in the frequency of babies' bowel movements. Decreased milk production and flow does not necessarily mean a slowdown in weight gain. We used to believe that decreased frequency of bowel movements was unusual, but likely normal for the exclusively breastfed baby since they often continued to gain weight well, at least for a while. Some babies would not have a bowel movement for a week at a time, sometimes longer. Practitioners generally believed that this was okay if babies were content and gaining weight. Some interpreted this infrequency of bowel movements as the baby's very efficient absorption of breastmilk from the intestinal tract. We no longer accept this as normal, but it is a relatively uncommon symptom, compared to the other symptoms.

## Mucousy or Bloody Bowel Movements

Bowel movements may become "mucousy" or greenish in color. Green, mucousy bowel movements were considered normal if everything else seemed okay, including the weight gain. Some babies will have droplets of blood in the bowel movements, which results in the "diagnosis" of an allergy to something in the breastmilk. This often happens after a period of days or weeks of mucousy bowel movements and indicates progression of the syndrome of late onset decreasing milk supply and flow. We cannot really explain adequately why a small minority of babies start having blood in the bowel movements. Typically, the blood is present only as little globules of blood in what is otherwise a relatively normal-looking bowel movement.

Our explanation for the blood in the bowel movements is that typically, the older baby (say 3 or 4 months of age) will drink at the breast if the flow is relatively rapid. Once the flow slows, many older babies will pull off the breast. The older baby may take the other breast, but again, pull off the breast before drinking much higher-fat milk. (Note: There is no definite "border" between low- and high-fat milk. The increase in fat is linear.) Thus, the baby may get two loads of relatively low-fat milk. Because fat content is relatively low, the stomach empties rapidly, with not only the breastmilk, but also gastric enzymes, such as pepsin as well as hydrochloric acid, which would not normally be found in the small intestine.

We do not have proof for this hypothesis, and it may not be true, but the presence of blood as small globules is not typical of large intestinal bleeding or the bleeding due to an anal fissure, for example. On the other hand, I (AP) have seen one baby whose blood in the stool was, in fact, different, with large amounts of bright red blood. However, even in this case the blood disappeared with treatment of late onset decreasing milk production and flow. Does this above explanation account for the blood? Maybe it is, as in the French expression *tirée par les cheveux* (pulled by the hair). Whatever the explanation, the blood disappears when the milk supply and flow are increased. It is important to re-emphasize, however, that slow or no weight gain, or even weight loss are late symptoms or signs of late onset decreasing milk supply and flow.

## Fussing and Pulling Away from the Breast

As mothers' milk supply and flow decreases, babies start pulling away from the breast, without always letting go of the breast, much to the mother's distress. As time goes on, babies become fussy and fussier while on the breast, pulling away earlier and earlier. Watch this video.

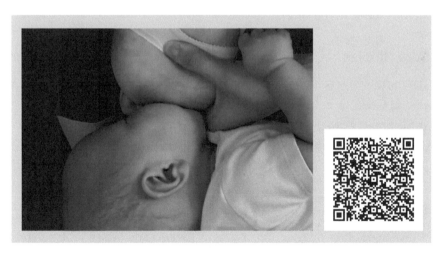

This video shows a baby of 2 months of age.

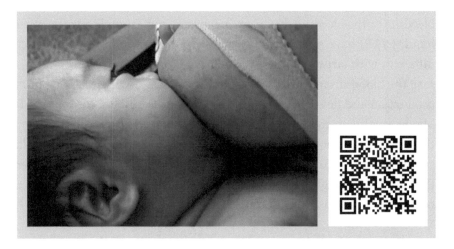

According to the mother, everything was fine until the 6-week routine postpartum follow-up. The mother was encouraged to take a combination birth control pill. Within 1 week, the baby, who was previously never fussy at the breast became fussy. The video shows the baby hardly drinking at all (no pauses in the chin).

## Sore Nipples

The mother starts having sore nipples, which she may not have had for several weeks or not at all. Nipple soreness can develop because of pulling at the breast as well as babies tending to slip down on to the nipple when the flow slows resulting in the baby sucking on the nipple, rather than on the breast.

## Sucking Fingers

When babies suck on their fingers, many parents and health professionals believe this is normal. We do not agree. We believe it is a common sign of late onset decreasing milk supply and flow. It explains why not all babies seem unhappy even though they are not getting as much milk from the breast. Also, these babies will accept a pacifier when they never did in the first few weeks and may suck on pacifiers for hours each day. If they continue to gain weight well, babies' fussiness is diagnosed as reflux or allergy to something in the mother's milk.

## Excessive Crying and "Colic"

If babies cry a lot, they get diagnosed with "colic." We do not believe that exclusively breastfed babies who are getting adequate milk from the breast get colic. If they are not getting enough milk, it's still not colic, whatever colic is. There is one proviso, however, and that is that some babies just want more milk than others of their weight and age. We have seen babies gaining plenty of weight, following their growth curve beautifully, who, when we increased the baby's intake of breastmilk stopped having "colic." Adults don't eat uniform amounts of food; neither do babies. Late onset decreasing milk supply and flow becomes most obvious around 2 to 3 months, the age when colic symptoms are supposed to diminish or stop.

## Breast Refusal

From the first days we started working with breastfeeding mothers, we heard about babies who suddenly stopped breastfeeding and went "on strike." Some babies preferred to suck their fingers rather than breastfeed. Typically, they continued night feedings, which may be why some continue to gain weight well. As time went on, however, some refused completely, especially if the mothers turned, in desperation, to expressed milk or formula by bottles. Why would this happen? After years of observing mothers and babies, we believe that it is due to decreased milk supply and flow.

## A Story of Late Onset Decreasing Milk Supply and Flow

Here is a typical story we hear frequently. This one came via email. I (JN) will copy the thread without changes. The baby is 3 months old and the mother emails to find out about whether it is okay to get the COVID-19 vaccine while breastfeeding. I answer that, "yes, it is good for you and for the baby." She also is concerned about the baby's slowing weight gain. The thread follows, exactly as we each wrote.

**JN**: As for the slowing of the weight gain. Your offering only one breast at a feeding would be a very good explanation for that. Click and read: http://ibconline.ca/one-side-or-two/ Feeding one side at a time and not offering the other breast often leads to a decrease in milk supply and fussiness of the baby, pulling at the breast, sucking his fingers. And very often to an incorrect diagnosis of "colic," "reflux," and/or "allergy to something in the mother's milk."

**Mother**: I think offering is incorrect (*sic*); he will only take one side. He doesn't want the 2nd side.

**JN**: If you change sides as he drinks less and less from the first side, before he is asleep, he will take the second side. Then how do you explain the slowing of the weight gain? Watch these videos: Really good drinking with English text, Twelve day old nibbling, English Text https://goo.gl/BeJZQn, "Borderline" drinking for video clips showing babies drinking well at the breast, or not. Watch the videos, read the texts, and then watch the videos again.

**Mother**: I was doing 2 sides, but he was having poops.

I presume she means, too many poops or green poops, I never asked because I did not want to get involved with color, frequency, pasty or liquidy, or whatever parents and doctors worry about with regards to bowel movements.

My doctor attributed it to too much foremilk and said to nurse longer per side. So doing 15 to 20 min per side and then he will only take the 2nd side just before bedtime (cluster feeding). He was gaining well until the 3 months weigh in. He has also been chewing at his hands, excessive drooling, and screaming when I try to get him to nurse the past couple days. The past week or more he nursed regularly every 2 hours. I have also started my period again, unsure if this affected my supply or milk.

**JN**: Nonsense about foremilk and hindmilk. I wish we had never heard of foremilk and hindmilk. The only result of this notion is babies starting not to gain weight properly.

The next step? You and your doctor will be concerned about the slow weight gain, you will be told to supplement with bottles of formula. And he will end up stopping breastfeeding.

What you describe is, exactly, late onset decreasing milk supply and flow. Click and read: http://ibconline.ca/decreased/

**Mother**: Yes, I was reading as I was writing! It all is making sense and suits the situation to a tee! Will start feeding both (not as long per side) as indicated, but is there anything else that can be done? Also, unsure if menstruation can affect supply or milk for babe. I breastfed my first child for 22 months and hope to do the same at least for this child. Thank you for your insight and the articles, I had perused the site but hadn't found this exact info. Also, I hadn't seen any info regarding covid-19 vaccine, so I appreciate that.

**Me**: So, your menstruation came back. It came back because your milk supply decreased, not because the menstruation resulted in your milk supply decreasing. This is a common myth that menstruation makes the milk supply decrease.

**Me**: P.S. You may require domperidone to bring back your milk supply even if you do start offering both breasts at each feeding. Things may have gone along too long. Click and read: Domperidone can increase the milk flow to the baby. Read carefully: http://ibconline.ca/domperidone/. We start with a dose of 30 mg (3 tablets) three times a day and often go up from there.

**End of thread**

This mother starts off, undoubtedly, with an abundant milk supply. She feeds her baby at both breasts at each feeding, but some "problem" with the baby's bowel movements causes the doctor to recommend she feed at only one breast at each feed. At first, *perhaps*, the bowel movements "improve" but soon, new problems arise. The weight gain slows, the baby becomes fussy.

## Prevention

As with any medical issue, prevention is much better than treatment. Preventing late onset decreased milk supply and flow starts at the beginning.

- Achieve the best latch possible as soon as possible after birth. If the baby has a tongue-tie, it should be released, preferably during the first day or two after birth when often a gentle push with a finger will release the tongue-tie.

- Teach the mother how to know a baby is drinking at the breast and not just sucking without drinking. *This is vital.*

- Show the mother how to use breast compressions, if necessary. We do not believe that breast compressions should be used *routinely*, but rather only when there is a need for the baby to receive more milk flow.

- Offer both breasts at each feeding. When the mother's milk supply is abundant, the baby may not take the second breast, but the mother should offer the second breast before the baby is fast asleep.

- Avoiding bottles and artificial nipples including pacifiers.

## Treatment

If late onset decreasing milk supply and flow has occurred, there are several specific steps mothers can take to increase their supply.

### Stop All Artificial Nipples

The first step is to stop all bottles and pacifiers. If the baby is older and receiving food pouches, these too may interfere with the baby's latch and may decrease the mother's milk supply and flow. Many cups for babies are not open cups at all, but essentially a different sort of bottle.

### Offer Both Breasts at Each Feeding

If the mother is offering only one breast at each feeding, have her offer both breasts at each feeding, starting immediately. Offering both breasts *may* be enough to turn things around if the situation has not deteriorated too much. Again, note that late onset decreasing milk supply and flow will *worsen* if *nothing* is done. Many mothers say that the baby will not take both breasts at each feeding; that the baby is "full" after the first side. Our lactation consultants rarely see this when these babies are breastfeeding in our presence. One reason the baby will not take the second side is that the mother keeps the baby on the first side until the baby is asleep, almost asleep, or lets go of the breast and sleeps. The baby will not seem interested in the second breast but may wake up and want to feed again in 1 to 2 hours. If the mother changes sides when the baby is no longer drinking even with compressions, and *before he begins to become too sleepy*, the baby almost always will take the second breast if offered.

## Stop Hormonal Contraception

If the mother is taking female hormones (usually the birth control pill, even the "minipill" and an IUD with progesterone), we strongly recommend she stop the hormones or have the IUD removed. (One exception would be a transgender female who should continue *physiological* doses of estrogen and progesterone.) Simply stopping the hormones, however, will not usually increase the milk supply and flow. These mothers will usually need domperidone to boost the milk supply.

## Get the Baby Back to the Breast

Usually, even if babies refuse the breast, they will take the breast again when they are asleep. We have had the occasional baby refuse the breast for days, being fed by bottle, until we could help the mother get the baby back to the breast. Of course, until we can see the mother and baby again, we would prefer the baby not be fed by bottle, but rather by open cup, but most of the mothers are just not comfortable with cup feeding a baby at this stage, though it is not usually complicated to cup feed a 4-month-old.

## Increase the Mother's Milk Supply and Milk Flow

Depending on the age of the baby and how fussy the baby is at the breast, partly based on history and how the baby breastfeeds at the clinic, our approach to treatment varies. In general, we want to increase the milk flow first.

### Domperidone

Domperidone increases the milk supply and flow of milk. We start with a dose of 30 mg (3 tablets) 3 times a day and sometimes go up from there. Our usual maximum dose is 160 mg/day, divided into 3 doses (6 tablets, 5 tablets, 5 tablets, total 16), though, in theory, 4 doses of 40 mg a day *might* be more effective. In the case of sleep-deprived new mothers, the fewer number of doses, perhaps, the better, as remembering to take pills several times a day risks forgetting a dose or two.

We treat the mother with domperidone for 7 to 14 days before releasing a tongue-tie if that was a precipitating factor in the decreased in milk flow. However, if the baby is younger than 3 months or so of age, we may do the tongue-tie release and start domperidone at the same time, since breast refusal after tongue-tie seems less common when the baby is younger.

Breast refusal after tongue-tie release is possible, even at 6 weeks of age, though much less common. It would have been ideal to release tongue-ties in hospital to prevent problems in the first place, but interestingly, very few of the babies we see with significant tongue-ties had the release at birth. Some with severe tongue-ties did not seem to have tongue-ties in the hospital. How odd.

## Conclusion

The diagnosis of late onset decreasing milk supply and flow is rarely made by pediatricians in Toronto and the mother's and baby's symptoms are typically misdiagnosed as colic, reflux, or allergy. When babies suddenly start pulling off or being fussy at the breast, sucking their fingers, and their weight gain slows, late onset decreasing supply and flow is often to blame. Practitioners can address these symptoms by increasing mothers' flow and supply.

CHAPTER 16

# Domperidone

Domperidone is a medication that effectively boosts milk supply and flow. Milk supply was not its original purpose but an interesting side effect. Domperidone is a peripheral dopamine antagonist that increases the release of prolactin from the pituitary and increases breastmilk production as a result. It works particularly well when mothers once had an abundant or very good milk supply, but the supply and flow decreased for some reason. Domperidone is extremely helpful for overcoming breastfeeding problems, particularly when the baby is not getting enough from the breast, but it is only *part of the approach* to making breastfeeding work. At the risk of tiresomely repeating ourselves, the earlier the initiation of treatment of breastfeeding problems, the better.

## Using Domperidone

Increasing milk supply and flow of milk is about more than prescribing domperidone. It is about overall good breastfeeding management: helping mothers latch the baby on as well as possible; knowing how well the baby drinks at the breast, offering both breasts at each feeding; and avoiding bottles. If supplementation is necessary, using a lactation aid at the breast does not undermine breastfeeding as much as a bottle.

## Dosage

Domperidone is especially helpful when used in conjunction with the techniques in the previous paragraph. In our clinic, we start with a dose of 30 mg (3 tablets) three times a day. Frequently we increase the dose in two steps, first to 40 mg three times a day, and then to 40 mg 4 times a day. On rare occasions, I (JN) have recommended the mother take up to 200 mg/day. We start with a lower dose to decrease the risk side effects, and to use the lowest dose that works.

## Timing of Medication

We used to say that it would be best to start domperidone only after the baby's age of 2 to 3 weeks, at a time when the prolactin levels in the mother's blood had basically bottomed out after being high during the pregnancy and immediately after birth. We have found, however, that the earlier domperidone is used, the more it increases milk supply and flow. Of course, we cannot be sure because we never just recommend domperidone and "off you go." Unfortunately, too often this is exactly what many doctors do: without watching the baby at the breast, without helping with the latch, or teaching mothers what they need to do to make sure the baby gets the maximum milk flow. Domperidone *alone* only occasionally works when the baby is not getting enough at the breast. It's only one part of the management of helping the baby get more milk.

Too often, doctors say to mothers, "Well, your baby is gaining well now, so you can stop the domperidone." If mothers are told to stop at an inappropriate time, milk supply *usually* decreases again, especially if the baby latches on poorly, the mother does not use breast compressions, she continues to feed on just one breast at a feeding or "block feeds," and the tongue-tie is not released. Furthermore, our *impression* is that when domperidone is stopped prematurely, mothers' supply does not always return to where it was on the same dose. We usually recommend the mother continue domperidone until babies are well established on food and will eat as much as they want if hungry. We do not know why this decreased responsiveness to domperidone occurs if stopped and restarted. In any case, it is an impression only.

## Tongue-Tie Release

Once the mother has been on domperidone for at least 1 week, we will do a tongue-tie release if there is one. There usually is. At this point, however, the situation may have improved to the point that the parents no longer want to do the tongue-tie release. We strongly encourage the parents to go forward with it, but the decision is theirs, after all. Tongue-tie, particularly if tight, may result in difficulty eating food, and difficulty in pronouncing certain sounds, especially the rolled "r."

## Stopping Domperidone

We usually recommend the mother continue the domperidone at least until the baby is eating food *well* and then wean from the domperidone very slowly, no more than one 10 mg tablet a week. Thus, if the mother is taking 3 tablets 3 times a day, it will take 9 weeks to wean off domperidone.

Why wean slowly? For two reasons: 1) When mothers stop domperidone too rapidly and too soon, the milk supply may decrease significantly, the baby becomes fussy at the breast, and may even refuse to latch on altogether. 2) Stopping the domperidone too quickly may result in anxiety, sleeplessness, depression in susceptible individuals, especially if the mother has been taking the domperidone for several months.

Regarding point 2, we have observed, after prescribing domperidone for more than 35 years, that most mothers do not experience anxiety, sleeplessness, and depression, but a small number do. Even though only small amounts cross the blood-brain barrier, domperidone may work as a mild antidepressant. If small amounts have been entering the brain over weeks and months, once the mother stops taking it, the domperidone will slowly leave the brain and go back into the general circulation. If mothers wean slowly off the medication, they usually will not have symptoms even if they are susceptible to depression. Keep in mind that many new mothers have postpartum depression and anxiety—even if they never took domperidone. Yet, when breastfeeding mothers are depressed or anxious, people are quick to blame domperidone.

Finally, we do not just hand out the domperidone prescriptions to all and sundry. We first help mothers improve how their babies latch on, which decreases her pain and helps babies get more milk from the breast. Domperidone is added to whatever else we do.

### When Babies Refuse the Breast

When babies refuse to latch on, even if mothers have a full supply, we use domperidone to increase the flow of milk. More milk means faster flow. Faster flow means that babies may be more willing to latch on to the breast. Once babies latch on at every feed, and they do it for a week or more, mothers can stop taking domperidone. We recommend that they don't stop "cold turkey," but rather wean themselves off the domperidone over 10 to 14 days.

## Possible Side Effects of Domperidone

In our experience, most side-effects occur in the first week or so and then disappear. These side-effects are usually mild and include headache, abdominal cramping, and diarrhea. Some mothers get dry mouth, but that is not as common.

### Diarrhea

Mothers with inflammatory bowel disease worry that domperidone will increase their symptoms, including diarrhea. Fortunately, most of our patients with inflammatory bowel disease have not had a problem with it.

### Migraines

However, domperidone can increase risk of more frequent and more severe headaches in mothers prone to migraines. This can be a real problem. Some decide to take additional medications to prevent and treat their migraines, including monoclonal antibodies (Diener et al., 2020). Some mothers decide not to take domperidone at all. We believe that increasing the success of breastfeeding *is* worth it, but we do not get migraines. If mothers need to stop taking domperidone, they can stop it relatively quickly because if the frequency and severity of migraines increases, they generally do so within the first 2 or 3 weeks after starting domperidone.

### Weight Gain

About 10% of people taking domperidone gain weight if they take it for more than a few weeks. The good news is that this weight gain is apparently due to fluid retention, and most mothers are reassured by this. When they stop taking domperidone, they lose the extra weight very quickly. However, some breastfeeding mothers eat more, feeling hungrier than usual, so the domperidone may not be the only thing causing them to gain weight.

## Most Doctors Do Not Know about Domperidone

If doctors have heard of domperidone, they are often leery about prescribing it. Honestly, we agree that doctors should be concerned about prescribing *any* unnecessary medication, even if the medications are usually helpful. All drugs potentially have side effects, some of which are quite serious. Take, for example, antibiotics. Antibiotics are frequently prescribed unnecessarily, even for obvious viral infections. They can cause death from anaphylaxis, and serious diarrhea from an overgrowth of *C. difficile*. Yet very few people seem to worry about overusing them. Given that, we are puzzled why doctors are so concerned about domperidone.

Doctors worry that domperidone can cause heart problems by prolonging the QTc interval on electrocardiogram (see the section on Domperidone Paranoia). Prolonged QTc intervals *may* cause fatal arrhythmia. They are most likely to occur in people over 60, not the usual age of breastfeeding mothers. Even in people over 60, it is a rare side effect. We agree that people over 60 should avoid domperidone. Domperidone is mostly used to treat reflux esophagitis, sometimes for eosinophilic esophagitis, and there are now safer drugs for these problems, such as proton pump inhibitors. If there is a family history of sudden, unexplained death in a young member of the mother's immediate family, it would be prudent to get an electrocardiogram before starting domperidone.

Interestingly, the SSRI class of antidepressants, and a wide range of other drugs, have the same effect of prolonging the QTc interval on electrocardiogram, yet doctors do not seem to worry about them. Other drugs which may prolong the QTc, include some antibiotics like azithromycin.

It's important to keep this in perspective. We have mothers in our clinic who take SSRIs (not prescribed by us), yet none have had to have an electrocardiogram before starting the antidepressant.

## Options for Domperidone

In some countries (USA, some EU countries), domperidone is difficult to get, but it not *illegal* to possess. Indeed, in the U.S., veterinarians have access to domperidone. Million-dollar racehorses with low milk supplies need treatment, but not human mothers. In Slovakia, physicians can prescribe domperidone for reflux (GERD), but not to increase milk supply.

Metoclopramide works like domperidone, but its side-effects are more worrisome. Metoclopramide drastically increases the risk of depression, so it is good to avoid for that reason alone (Hale, Kendall-Tackett, & Cong, 2018). A rare but serious side-effect of metoclopramide is tardive dyskinesia. Metoclopramide passes the blood-brain barrier in greater amounts than domperidone.

Sulpiride also increases milk supply and flow and is a favorite in South Africa. It is an antidepressant with all the possible side effects of SSRI but is not available in the U.S. or Canada. Interestingly, sertraline (Zoloft) also increases milk supply. We do not recommend sulpiride, or other SSRI antidepressants for increasing milk supply as they can have many unwanted side-effects, especially if used long term.

## Domperidone Paranoia

This topic needs a section on its own. Domperidone is a very useful medication that people malign and describe as extremely dangerous. However, the side-effect profile of domperidone is much safer than it is for many other drugs that doctors prescribe for new mothers.

### Domperidone and Cardiac Arrhythmias

Domperidone was banned in the U.S. because some very ill cancer patients developed fatal cardiac arrhythmias after being treated with domperidone to prevent nausea and vomiting caused by anti-cancer medication. These patients were receiving *extremely high doses of domperidone intravenously* every few hours. Breastfeeding mothers take it *orally* and in much smaller amounts. A single IV dose given to the cancer patient is what a breast-feeding mother would take for an entire day. Furthermore, only about 13% to 17% of an *oral* dose of domperidone is absorbed from the intestinal tract, compared to 100% given intravenously. On top of this, domperidone may not even be the culprit. Many cancer drugs can cause serious arrythmia by decreasing or increasing serum potassium. Unfortunately, even with all this qualifying information, doctors still believe that domperidone is dangerous and will not it prescribe to breastfeeding women. Their attitude seems to be, "Better a live formula-feeding mother than a dead breastfeeding mother."

This fear can also spread to patients. We have clients who are initially enthusiastic but are afraid after they've been online. What sticks in their mind is, "fatal cardiac arrhythmias." Not a surprise, is it? When we went online, this is what we found under, "People also ask." The question was, "who should not take domperidone"? Answer:

Domperidone *products are contraindicated in patients with severe hepatic impairment, conditions where cardiac conduction is, or* could be, impaired or where there is underlying cardiac disease such as conges-tive heart failure, and when co-administered with QT-prolonging medicines or potent CYP3A4 inhibitors. (Apr 25, 2014).

Most drugs would receive a write-up like that. Another question asks, "How safe is domperidone?" Answer:

It is already known that domperidone *can cause irregular heartbeats* (heart arrhythmia). A recent review of the safety and effectiveness of domperidone found that it may slightly increase the risk of an irregular heartbeat and death due to heart problems.

When parents read up on domperidone, who would ignore a word like "death"? We do not prescribe domperidone if mothers are at risk for sudden unexpected death or they have a strong family history of it without first doing an electrocardiogram to rule out a prolonged QTc interval. Even then, not all unexpected sudden deaths in young people are due to prolonged QTc on electrocardiograms.

## Our Response to the Health Canada Warnings

Health Canada issued a warning about domperidone that was based on two studies published in 2010. Both were secondary analyses of databases from the Netherlands (van Noord, Dieleman, van Herpen, Verhamme, & Sturkenboom, 2010) and Saskatchewan (Johannes, Varas-Lorenzo, McQuay, Midkiff, & Fife, 2010). The populations in these studies were older adults, thus not generalizable to breastfeeding mothers. The average age of the patients was 72.5 in one study (van Noord et al., 2010) and 79.4 in the other (Johannes et al., 2010). Many patients already had health problems, such as high blood pressure, coronary artery disease, and congestive heart failure. Neither study demonstrated that domperidone *caused* any adverse health effects.

Interestingly, further analysis of one of these studies found that younger patients who took domperidone had a risk of cardiac problems that was near zero (Johannes et al., 2010). Women's risk of heart problems was lower than men's, as was true for patients who had been on domperidone longer (Johannes et al., 2010). All these findings should reassure breastfeeding mothers or those who prescribe medication for them.

### Warning about Higher Doses

Health Canada's warning about doses higher than 30 mg per day was based on the second study (van Noord et al., 2010). Out of the 1,304 deaths, only 10 patients were taking domperidone. Of the 10 taking domperidone, only four took more than 30 mg per day. These patients were older and sicker than the population of breastfeeding mothers. *Health Canada's warning came from FOUR ill, older patients.*

Domperidone is, or was generally used to treat gastrointestinal problems, such as acid reflux. Symptoms of heart disease may mimic symptoms of a gastrointestinal illness. It is possible that some of the patients taking domperidone may have thought they had a gastrointestinal problem when they really had a heart problem. While the authors attempted to account for this possible protopathic bias, it was hard to tease out (van Noord et al., 2010). Furthermore, because domperidone is, or was available over the counter in parts of Europe when these studies were done, some of the patients in the study may have been self-medicating, so their dosage may have been even higher. The study only asked about prescriptions for domperidone, not over-the-counter use, possibly skewing the results. The study also did not provide data on key health indicators, as smoking and use of non-prescription drugs (Johannes et al., 2010).

We do not believe that this data is strong enough to make a recommendation of using a dose of domperidone of only 10 mg (1 pill) three times a day. A dose of 30 mg per day is not effective for breastfeeding issues. Interestingly, the authors did not tell physicians to avoid higher doses. Rather, they said that certain patients (i.e., at risk for sudden cardiac death) should avoid domperidone. We agree with that recommendation.

## Risk Associated with Domperidone vs. Birth Control Pills

Contrast Health Canada's reaction to domperidone vs. their reaction to birth control pills. Several women in Europe and North America have died taking birth control pills (and 23 in Canada over 8 years). Birth control pills increase risk for venous thromboembolism (Dunn, 2009). People think that birth control pills are worth the risk. This is odd considering that there are safer methods of contraception. Yet, we cannot use domperidone to improve breastfeeding success because it is "dangerous."

When all is said and done, if physicians consider something important, like preventing pregnancy, they will weigh the risks against the benefits. If the benefits outweigh the risks, they will prescribe the birth control pill because preventing pregnancy outweighs the very small risk of thromboembolism, which can be fatal. On the other hand, in the mind of many health professionals, breastfeeding is not important enough, though the risks of not breastfeeding, including shortened lifespan in both the mother and the child, documented elsewhere in this book, are just not worth the tiny risk of domperidone. Perhaps this is an unfair comment, since most health professionals just do not know about the risks of not breastfeeding, or do not believe that there are risks.

## Conclusion

Breastfeeding mothers using domperidone are generally younger, healthy females. They do not belong to the same demographic group as the patients in the studies. Furthermore, the caution about higher doses of domperidone stems from one study with only four patients on higher doses. In our opinion, Health Canada's warning about higher doses is an overreaction. Finally, considering the limitations of these studies as outlined above, there is no evidence that domperidone causes ventricular arrhythmias or sudden cardiac death in younger women. Only if there is a history of sudden unexpected death in a close family member, should an electrocardiogram be done to rule out a prolonged QTc interval which is what is associated with sudden unexpected death. If the QTc interval is normal, domperidone does not cause heart problems, specifically sudden death.

# CHAPTER 17

# Relactation

In an ideal world, relactation would never be necessary. Unfortunately, some women need to relactate, often because a health professionals sabotaged their breastfeeding by telling them to stop when it wasn't necessary. Family and friends also often undermine the mother's breastfeeding. When babies are taken off the breast and fed by bottle, even with expressed breastmilk, they may refuse to latch on again. Hence the need to re-establish breastfeeding.

## Why Are Mothers Unnecessarily Told to Stop Breastfeeding?

### Medications

Health professionals may tell mothers to stop breastfeeding so that they can take a medication. As most medications are prescribed for several days, it may be difficult to restart breastfeeding while maintaining the milk supply. In fact, few medications require mothers to interrupt breastfeeding. Often there is a safe substitute medication available for a drug that is truly contraindicated during breastfeeding.

### Lower Weight Gain

If the baby's weight is lower than expected, in many cases, supplementation is not needed, especially if supportive intervention is started early. A mother needs timely help to improve her breastfeeding. If a supplement is truly necessary, she can use a lactation aid at the breast and domperidone to increase milk production and flow. Unfortunately, many mothers are told to supplement with 3 ounces of formula at each feeding, for example. This frequently leads to breast refusal, and eventually, the baby receives mostly or only formula.

### Mishandling Sore Nipples

Taking the baby off the breast, or recommending a nipple shield, may result in the baby refusing the breast altogether. A baby on a nipple shield is, essentially, off the breast. In both cases, the milk supply decreases so that the baby is even less likely to take the breast after the nipples heal.

### Inappropriate Custody Arrangements

Some parents of young breastfeeding babies are given inappropriate overnight access in custody disputes. When these babies come back to their mothers, they may refuse the breast. Older babies may spend nights away from the breast, crying constantly.

## What Can Be Done?

The best-case scenario is to prevent breastfeeding problems from Day 1 of the baby's life. Furthermore, the earlier breastfeeding problems are addressed, say within the first 2 or so weeks after birth, the easier they are to deal with.

### If the Baby Still Latches on to the Breast

If more difficult problems arise, it is good if the baby still latches on to the breast. The mother breastfeeds and supplements, if necessary, using a lactation aid at the breast. She follows the approach we describe throughout this book to increase the baby's breastmilk intake. If the baby still requires supplementation at about 4 months of age, the baby can be supplemented with food, which many mothers prefer over bottles, formula, and even (unfortunately) the lactation aid, which many find difficult to use. However, with practice, it often becomes easy. Domperidone is also very useful in this situation.

Many doctors warn mothers about not starting food before 6 months of age, based on the recommendations of the WHO or their own country's pediatric society. If everything is going along fine with the breastfeeding, we agree. Babies should start food when they are showing obvious readiness (trying to grab food out of the parent's plate). On the other hand, if the baby is being supplemented with bottles of formula, starting food will usually get the baby off the bottle. Food can even be started by 4 months of age, sometimes even earlier. And formula, or better, breastmilk, can be added to the food. It was not that long ago that pediatric societies around the world recommended starting food at 4 months of age.

## Increase Food Intake

The baby in this video was still breastfeeding, but the mother wanted to stop using the lactation aid to supplement her 4-month-old baby. She was tired of using it. Food allowed her to stop the lactation aid without giving bottles. How much food could babies receive? As much as they wanted, as frequently as they would eat the food without being forced.

Mother's milk or formula (she was using formula in the lactation aid), could be added to the food. Oil such as vegetable oil or olive oil can be added to the food to increase the caloric content of food. At 4 months of age, parents are reluctant to give "pieces" of food, so we recommend purees (made by the parents) at first. Easy foods to start with are avocado (a bit on the pricey side in Canada) or banana. However, by 5 months age, babies can handle pieces of food to chew on. The baby may even have a tooth or two. (See Chapter 21 on Starting Babies on Food.)

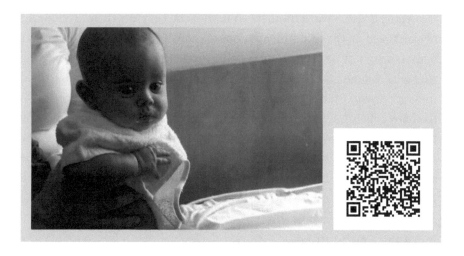

## If the Baby No Longer Takes the Breast

The first step is to increase the mother's milk supply and especially the flow of milk from the breast. Thus, we recommend that she express her milk and take domperidone to increase her milk supply. The more milk the mother produces, the more likely the baby will start latching on.

## Alternate Feeding Methods

Methods of feeding, other than bottles, should be used to feed the baby breastmilk or formula (if necessary). The idea is to increase the likelihood that babies will return to the breast.

### Cup Feeding

Even small premature babies can drink from an open cup. Full-term 3-month-olds should be able to do the same. A young baby can also feed well from a spoon, though obviously this may take more time.

### Finger Feeding

Finger feeding is *not* a good way to feed a baby a complete meal, in our opinion, but can be used to get the baby to take the breast. In this video, the baby has never taken the breast. He was born 2 months prematurely. As so often happens in our NICUs, the baby and mother were given no breastfeeding help in the hospital. We decided to do the video to show how finger feeding works to help the baby latch on. Finger feeding was used to prepare the baby to take the breast by taking the edge off his hunger so that he was more patient at the breast. Milk flow helps the baby to latch on and drink at the breast. The baby in this video is 2 months old and exclusively breastmilk fed.

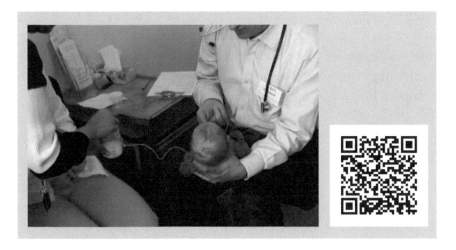

I (JN) finger feed the baby for 30 to 60 seconds or so, then moved the baby to the right breast. The baby did not take the right breast because he had already fed well on that side. With the second attempt to latch the baby on the right breast, the breast was less "full" and the flow of milk slower, even with the lactation aid at the breast. After trying three times on the right breast, we moved the baby over to the left breast. After a couple of tries, the baby took the breast and breastfed well, with the lactation aid at the breast helping with the flow.

## Babywearing and Domperidone

The mother should "wear" the baby with the breast exposed in such a way that the baby will be able to find the breast and latch on. We recommend domperidone even when mothers are producing more than enough milk to feed their babies. More milk still, greater flow, making it more likely the baby will latch on.

## Conclusion

Sometimes, usually through mismanagement, mothers' milk supply and flow drops, and babies may refuse to latch on. Or the mother was told, usually wrongly, that she should not breastfeed. Or some mothers decide to stop breastfeeding but change their minds. The first step is to increase mothers' supply and flow. When supply increases, babies are more likely to latch on. A lactation aid may be necessary to increase the flow until the mothers' supply increases. While relactating, mothers should use alternative feeding methods so that they can avoid bottles. If babies are older than 4 months, they can also be supplemented with food rather than formula.

# CHAPTER 18

# Inducing Lactation

We will, in this discussion, refer to the "person" wishing to induce lactation, since it is not only women who induce lactation but also trans women and we have worked with a few men who wished to induce lactation. Why would a person want to induce lactation? The possible reasons are legion. We will list the reasons that we have heard from people coming to the clinic or who have contacted us through our website.

## Reasons for Inducing Lactation

### Having a Baby Through a Gestational Carrier

Amongst people attending our clinic, one of the most common reasons for inducing lactation is that a person is having a baby through a gestational carrier. Or, the baby is not genetically related to the adopting person, but the adopting parent would like to breastfeed the baby. Why would that person want to breastfeed? We have never studied this question, or even asked the person inducing lactation why they would want to breastfeed. We assume that all parents-to-be want the best for the baby and that they know that breastfeeding is the best for their baby. Furthermore, when that person will be a parent, the adopting person often wishes to take a "physical" part, sharing their body in raising the baby, when they could not, usually, give birth themselves.

### Adoption

On occasion, a woman (we have never been asked this by a man), would like to induce lactation for a baby she will adopt, but there is not yet a baby to be adopted. Although we understand the desire for the woman to prepare as long as possible beforehand, we are concerned about having someone on our protocol, including the use of female hormones, for more than the length of a normal pregnancy.

### Co-Lactation

Another common situation is that the parents are both women, one of whom is pregnant and plans to breastfeed, and the other would like to be involved in the care of the baby, including helping to breastfeed the baby. This may be to ensure the baby can be exclusively breastfed, and also to share the breastfeeding and for both parents to enjoy breastfeeding. In a few cases, in addition to the above-mentioned reason, the pregnant partner was having twins and the non-pregnant partner wanted to ensure that both babies were exclusively breastfed. That situation is even more relevant if one partner is pregnant with triplets.

### Sexual Play

We have had a few inquiries from male/female couples, the female of which wishes to induce lactation so that milk production by the woman can become part of the couple's sexual play and relationship. We do not judge what people do in private, but we are concerned about prescribing medication for this reason and have never agreed to do so. Perhaps we are old fashioned. (Perhaps a female/female couple might also wish to induce lactation for this reason, but we have never been approached for this reason, at least not that we know of).

## How to Induce Lactation

To induce lactation, we prescribe medication so that the person's body "thinks" that they are pregnant. Several hormones are made, both in the pituitary gland and in the placenta during pregnancy, that prepare the mother's body to sustain the pregnancy and to make milk. In a typical pregnancy, the mother starts to produce milk at about 16 to 17 weeks gestation.

We try to duplicate, as much as possible, the hormonal milieu that occurs in the mother and fetus during pregnancy. However, the endocrinology of pregnancy is extremely complex, and it is important to accept that duplicating it exactly, is probably not possible, or at least not yet in 2022. We can only, practically, treat the mother with estrogen, progesterone, and domperidone, which increases the prolactin level. Other hormones can be given, but need to be given by injection, probably daily, which is not very practical. Even that would not duplicate the hormonal variations during pregnancy. Since milk production in pregnant women starts about 16 to 17 weeks after implantation of the ovum, we decided that a person inducing lactation should follow our protocol for at least 4 months (16 to 17 weeks) before the baby is born.

We should mention that there are stories of people who induced lactation by just pumping their breasts in anticipation of a baby's birth. Or they simply put the baby to their breasts and produced milk, even sufficient milk to exclusively breastfeed a newborn baby. We doubt the reliability of these stories but accept that nothing is impossible. Were these people who just recently stopped breastfeeding a child? Or could they have had a prolactinoma (a benign tumor of the pituitary gland) that resulted in significant milk production? Who knows? And we have never spoken to any person(s) who reputedly did this.

## Medications We Recommend for Inducing Lactation

### A Combination Pill Containing Estrogen and Progesterone, With a Relatively Higher Dose of Progesterone

Most people taking this combination will simply take a birth control pill. Some say that a higher relative amount of progesterone is more effective, but we could find no studies to confirm this. It is, of course, possible to take the hormones in separate amounts, but the more pills one takes, the greater the risks of missing or mistaking doses.

To "simulate" pregnancy, the person inducing lactation should not take the "placebo" pills that are in the package for preventing pregnancy and they should skip from the last "active" pill to the next "active" pill for the "next" month.

The person inducing lactation continues with the pill until approximately 6 to 8 weeks before the baby is to be born. The reason for this is to give sufficient time to build up the milk supply before the baby is born so that the baby will breastfeed and be able to receive milk from the breast. If milk flows, the baby is more likely to latch on and breastfeed.

### Domperidone

In addition to the two hormones, we treat the person with domperidone, at a starting dose of 3 tablets 3 times a day starting at the same time as the hormones. We start at this dose which can be increased if necessary. However, as long as the person inducing lactation is on the combination pill, it is unlikely they will produce much milk, just as a pregnant woman will not produce a lot of milk during the pregnancy.

## Six to 8 Weeks Before the Baby Is Due

The person inducing lactation stops the estrogen and progesterone at this time. This, if the person is a woman, will result in uterine and thus vaginal bleeding, perhaps a fairly heavy bleed. If bleeding is very heavy or prolonged (for a lot more than a typical menstrual period), she should consult with her doctor or gynecologist to make sure that there is no pathological cause. This is also true if she has significant bleeding during the induction period, when no bleeding should occur because of the hormones she is taking.

At this point, having stopped the hormones, (but *not* the domperidone, which they will have to take, probably, the entire time of breastfeeding), the person inducing lactation, should start expressing/pumping her/his breasts to start increasing the milk supply and flow. In theory, milk expression should be done 8 to 10 times a day, essentially as often as the baby would be breastfeeding. Of course, this may not be practical if the person inducing lactation works at a job with no privacy. Several persons inducing lactation with us have been loath to let their co-workers know they were inducing lactation. Furthermore, they may not have enough time to express or pump during the usual breaks available. This problem can be partially alleviated by more frequent expression at home in the evenings or weekends.

The person inducing lactation should not expect much milk at first, just as a pregnant woman would not necessarily expect a lot of milk if she expressed milk 6 to 8 weeks before the baby is born. Yet she may produce plenty of milk once the baby is born. Likewise, the person inducing lactation may see a definite steady increase in the amount of milk they can pump over time. (We have stated this frequently throughout this book: what a mother can pump and what the baby receives from the breast are not necessarily the same. A baby well latched on will get more than the breastfeeding person can pump; a baby poorly latched on will get less.)

## When To Put the Baby to the Breast

The sooner the baby goes to the breast, the better. Immediately after birth is ideal. In some jurisdictions, the person inducing lactation can be in the delivery room to immediately put the baby to the breast. In other jurisdictions, this may not be possible. In fact, in some jurisdictions, the person inducing lactation may not be able to have the baby for 3 weeks or more after birth, in order to allow the birth mother to change her mind about not keeping the baby.

This possibility needs to be kept in mind. If the baby is bottle-fed for 3 weeks before the person inducing lactation can breastfeed, the baby may not take the breast. What to do? It's not easy. The best option would be for the birth mother to breastfeed the baby until the person inducing lactation has the right to take the baby. Or the birth mother gives up the baby sooner, with the proviso that the birth mother can change her mind about keeping the baby. This situation can be emotionally difficult for everyone.

On the other hand, if this is a situation where the woman giving birth has contracted to be the gestational carrier for the parents to be, with a fertilized egg, which comes either from the one partner (egg from one parent, fertilized by the other, or egg from one parent fertilized by donated sperm, or donated egg, fertilized by the other parent), there should be no issue, and the baby is handed over to the parents as soon as is practical, one hopes within the first hour or two after birth or a few days at the most. This should be specified in the contract.

## Should the Birth Mother Breastfeed?

Yes, we think this would be ideal, at least from the point of view of the baby and the person who will be the parent. Of course, not all birth mothers will agree, especially if the pregnancy was unwanted. Nevertheless, in some of the situations where we have helped mothers induce lactation, the birth mother was happy to breastfeed for the first few days and some even continued to pump their milk for the baby for several weeks.

The concern is that if the birth mother breastfeeds, she may deeply regret giving up the baby. Of course, she might still regret it even if she does not breastfeed. If the birth mother was a gestational carrier and had signed a contract, she may be sad to give up the baby, though legally, she might not have a choice. Breastfeeding the baby may cause her even more distress than she expected. On the other hand, we have been involved with, and have also heard of situations where the birth mother wanted to breastfeed, was delighted to breastfeed so that the baby will get the best start in life. Some women become gestational carriers out of pure selflessness, doing something wonderful for people that is a gift for life.

On the other hand, if the pregnancy was unwanted, breastfeeding may cause the birth mother to change her mind and keep her baby. We have no information on how often this happens, but as unhappy as this result would be for the adopting parents, a pregnant woman who is not a gestational carrier should have the right to change her mind.

If the birth mother is a gestational carrier, as far as we know, breastfeeding did not result in her trying to keep the baby, at least not in any case where we were involved in helping a person inducing lactation to breastfeed.

## When the Parents Are Two Women and One Is Pregnant

In this situation, the person inducing lactation has more time to build up the milk supply before it is necessary to feed the baby on the breast. Of course, there is no harm in putting the baby to the breast "for practice" and get the baby used to both parents, but the initial feedings should really be done by the birth mother. The mother who was pregnant needs to get off to the best start possible, with breastfeeding going well (no soreness, baby is getting plenty of milk from the breast and does not need supplementation). In such a case, we would recommend that the person inducing lactation has more time to build up the milk supply, keeping the baby exclusively breastfeeding on the birth mother to, say, at least 4 weeks after birth. This "4 weeks" is a guess; we don't really know.

## Follow-Up

We try to follow up with all our patients inducing lactation, just as we would any parent/baby pair who may be having difficulty breastfeeding. Just because the situation is one of induced lactation, does not mean the mother may not have sore nipples, though we would hope that doesn't happen if we were advising the mother before the birth. Nevertheless, photos and videos of what is a good latch are not the same as having a real baby in one's arms and trying to latch a baby on well. In our experience, most persons inducing lactation do *not* produce all the milk the baby requires and are obliged to supplement the baby. On the other hand, if there are two people breastfeeding one baby, that may work out.

Ideally, any supplement given to the baby would be donated breastmilk, same as with any mother who may not be producing enough milk. Breastmilk can be obtained from breastfeeding friends or relatives or, in some cases, from breastmilk banks. Though, because most human milk banks reserve their donated milk for premature babies or for babies who cannot tolerate formula, it is unlikely the mother of a healthy full-term baby will be able to obtain breastmilk from a milk bank.

There are websites that match breastfeeding mothers with parents who need breastmilk for the baby. A good site will go through the requirements for the donating mother to follow to make sure the milk is safe; that is, no evidence of possible infection that might pass through the milk (negative tests for HIV, HTLV virus and other infections that might be passed to the baby). See the section on maternal infections and breastfeeding. It is necessary to state that there be *no* monetary compensation for the donated (by definition) breastmilk. When there is money involved, corruption is always possible, including adding formula or cows' milk to the breastmilk to increase the amount.

We do not agree that donors need to avoid taking all medications. Most medication enters the milk in insignificant amounts or none at all. Does a tiny amount of drug for high blood pressure, or to treat hypothyroidism make the donator's milk less acceptable than formula? If it is the usual situation of a breastfeeding mother being able to take medication and continue breastfeeding because the benefits of breast-feeding outweigh the risks of not breastfeeding, then why reject the milk of a mother taking the same medication?

It is also important that the person donating the milk be reasonably close geographically to the person receiving the milk so that milk can be donated "face to face." Depending on the post office, or even delivery services, may not get the milk to the breastfeeding parent in time, dry ice or not.

## Case Study

One day, I (JN) received a phone call from a mother who wanted to breast-feed a baby whom she just found out was available to adopt. The baby was to be born in a week. We discussed what could be done. She had breastfed a previous baby, born to her, for 18 months without problems, but since then, was not able to get pregnant despite trying everything. The cause of her inability to become pregnant was not diagnosed.

After a discussion, I prescribed domperidone 30 mg three times a day for her and as well she had started taking some sort of mother's milk tea. I asked her to come to the clinic as soon as possible after she received the baby.

She came to the clinic with the baby at 2 weeks of age. The baby was exclusively breastfeeding. According to *our* scale the baby, born at term at a good weight, was 250 grams (1/2 pound) below birthweight. *Yet, he was drinking very well at the breast.* I was reassured by how well he was drinking and also reassured the mother, but I admit, I was worried.

I asked the mother to continue as she was doing and asked her to return in a week. A week after the first visit the baby had gained 200 grams (about 7 ounces). *Still more importantly,* the baby was drinking very well at the breast.

The mother breastfed the baby exclusively to 6 months of age and continued breastfeeding him with added food until 18 months of age. The photos below show the baby at 3 months of age, exclusively breastfeeding, and then again at 6 months of age when he was just starting food.

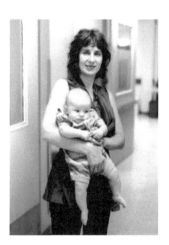 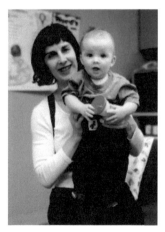

This is a very happy result. Happily, this was the very first mother and baby I ever helped induce lactation (although, really, all I did was prescribe domperidone and give reassurance). Nevertheless, it encouraged me to look more at this possibility of inducing lactation.

# MOTHERS' HEALTH

# CHAPTER 19

# When Mothers Are Sick

Many health professionals assume that mothers cannot breastfeed if they have an infectious disease. This belief spawned many of the draconian policies restricting mother and baby contact during COVID-19. However, health professionals should know that for most infectious diseases, breast-feeding protects babies rather than put them at risk. This has been amply demonstrated during the COVID-19 pandemic.

## Infectious Diseases

Most infectious diseases, particularly viral infections, are contagious for days, even weeks before the mother knows that she is sick. Thus, their babies have already been exposed and likely infectious themselves before mothers know they are. For example, chicken pox has an incubation period of 10 to 21 days. During that time, mothers are generally asymptomatic, but they can infect others through close contact. Even though babies have already been exposed, many health professionals tell mothers to stop breastfeeding. Such advice makes no sense. Breastfeeding works side-by-side with a baby's own immune system, such as it is (not very developed yet if the baby is younger than 6 months), to protect babies from becoming sick. It is the best of all situations. The baby becomes immune to the sickness, but not the infection. Fair enough. Occasionally, the baby may manifest signs of infection, but almost always, the baby is mildly sick, not seriously so.

A baby's first line of defense are the linings of their bodies, such as the skin and linings of the gastrointestinal and respiratory tracts. Mucus covers the intestinal lining and respiratory lining, which helps prevents contact between them and bacteria and viruses. In addition, Paneth cells in the intestinal lining produce and secrete antimicrobial peptides. These peptides shape the composition of the microbiome. Breastfeeding's protective molecules complement the baby's own immune system (Cacho & Lawrence, 2017).

## Breastfeeding Protects Babies Against Infection

Oligosaccharides in human milk protect babies by binding to pathogenic organisms and establishing the microbiome in the intestinal tract. Also, gangliosides, mucins, and glycoproteins all bind to potentially pathogenic pathogens, including HIV, rotavirus, *Escherichia coli*, and Salmonella. As Cacho and Lawrence (2017) note, lactoferrin is an example of a breastmilk glycoprotein that protects babies against infection, and there are many others.

> Lactadherin can inactivate viruses and limits inflammation by increasing the effective phagocytosis of apoptotic cells... The list of bioactive glycoproteins in human milk is still expanding, and their individual multifunctional nature is just being described. Butyrophilin, leptin, adiponectin, bile salt-stimulated lipase lysozyme, lactoperoxidase (LP), xanthine dehydrogenase, α-lactalbumin, κ-casein, and β-casein are just a few of these glycoproteins requiring additional study (p.2).

Breastmilk also contains large numbers of macrophages which phagocytize (eat) harmful bacteria without initiating an inflammatory response. The inflammatory response can damage tissues, so that the presence of these macrophages is an important adaptive response to diminishing possible harm from the immune response itself.

The antibodies (also called immunoglobulins) present in breastmilk are mostly of the secretory IgA type, representing over 90% of the immunoglobulins in milk. Secretory IgA molecules bind to bacteria and prevent their ability to cause infection. As with macrophages, sIgA does not cause an inflammatory response, which, to repeat, is important, given the huge numbers of bacteria in infants' intestinal tract and the potential damage that inflammation can cause.

Even with all the things that we know protect breastfeeding babies, healthcare providers still think that babies need to be separated from their mothers when they are sick. In most cases, this is not only unnecessary, but undesirable. Below is a listing of common infectious diseases listed in alphabetic order.

## Common Infectious Diseases and Breastfeeding

Some diseases, such as COVID-19 and HIV, at first, received a great deal of attention. In the case of COVID-19, there were strict recommendations to avoid close contact between mother and baby. As a result, these policies obstructed breastfeeding. However, subsequent research demonstrated that stopping breastfeeding was neither necessary nor desirable, certainly not with COVID-19. It is typical of the thinking of some government agencies that "breastfeeding is unsafe until proved otherwise."

The situation with HIV was more complicated until medications were developed that protected mothers and their babies during the pregnancy and breastfeeding. Now recommendations with regard to breastfeeding when women are infected with HIV have changed.

Besides increasing the risk of infection for infants, mother-baby separation may have another unintended consequence: interfering with attachment. According to Tran and colleagues (2020), interference with bonding can have lifelong consequences for both mother and baby. Routine separation is not only not necessary, but it also violates "first do no harm."

### Brucellosis

Brucellosis is an infection transmitted from infected domesticated animals (cows, pigs, sheep, and goats) to humans. People can be infected through their damaged skin, or by eating the improperly cooked meat, or drinking unpasteurized milk of these animals. It occurs wherever humans raise animals for meat and milk. People who work with livestock (e.g., farmers or veterinarians) are at higher risk of infection.

Doxycycline, rifampicin, cotrimoxazole/sulphamethoxazole, and ciprofloxacin are amongst the antibiotics used to treat brucellosis. Since the bacterium of brucellosis can be transmitted through mothers' milk, we would recommend treating both mother and baby simultaneously for an adequate period of time. There is no need to interrupt breastfeeding. Doxycycline is no longer considered contraindicated in breastfeeding (Todd et al., 2015). Practitioners assumed that doxycycline was a problem because it would stain and weaken children's teeth like tetracycline, a related, similar type of antibiotic. However, doxycycline does not damage teeth even when given to young children directly.

## COVID-19

Whenever a new virus appears, health professionals' first instinct is to tell mothers not to breastfeed. This certainly happened with COVID-19. The Centers for Disease Control and Prevention in the U.S. immediately recommended separation of the mother and baby if the mother had actual, or even suspected infection. Fortunately, World Health Organization recommended that breastfeeding not be interrupted, and that mothers and babies not be separated. The following are quoted from the World Health Organization:

> ...that mothers with suspected or confirmed COVID-19 should be encouraged to initiate or continue to breastfeed. Mothers should be counselled that the benefits of breastfeeding substantially outweigh the potential risks for transmission.

> Mother and infant should be enabled to remain together while rooming-in throughout the day and night and to practice skin-to-skin contact, including Kangaroo Mother Care, especially immediately after birth and during establishment of breastfeeding, whether they or their infants have suspected or confirmed COVID-19 (World Health Organization, 2020).

The Canadian Paediatric Society made a similar statement (Narvey & Canadian Paediatric Society Fetus and Newborn Committee, 2021).

Mothers being investigated for or found to be positive with COVID-19 infection should not be separated from their infants. Rooming in should occur after a discussion of risks and benefits, thereby allowing for shared decision-making with families and their healthcare providers. There is some evidence to suggest that infants can be infected with SARS-CoV-2 postnatally. Preventing postnatal infection should focus on enhanced hygiene to limit risk for transmission.

Mothers should practice skin-to-skin care and breastfeed while in hospital, with some modifications to usual processes. Among these precautions, mothers should practice meticulous hand hygiene, don a surgical/procedure mask when within 2 metres of their infant, and practice hand hygiene before skin-to-skin contact, breastfeeding, and routine infant care. Mother and infant should be discharged home as soon as they are deemed ready and convalesce at home in accordance with hospital guidance and local public health recommendations.

Not surprisingly, breastmilk neutralized COVID and produced anti-COVID immune factors (IgA and IgG). A study of 18 milk samples from COVID+ women found that their milk did not contain SARS-CoV-2 RNA (Pace et al., 2021). In addition, they found that:

> … milk produced by infected mothers is a source of anti-SARS-CoV-2 IgA and IgG and neutralizes SARS-CoV-2 activity. These results support recommendations to continue breastfeeding during mild to moderate maternal COVID-19 illness as milk likely provides specific immunologic benefits to infants (p. 1).

### Is that not like a vaccine?

We should also remember that some infections may transmit in utero, but the mother's body may protect her baby. A study of 42 pregnant women with COVID-19 found that none of the babies were born infected (Marin-Gabriel et al., 2020). If mothers are infected after the birth, it may be days before they have symptoms. Thus, their babies have already been exposed, and if the baby is breastfeeding, they are protected against serious disease.

If treatment is available, mother and baby should be treated together, and breastfeeding should continue. Breastfeeding also prevents vertical transmission of the virus from mother to baby (Tran et al., 2020). This study of 101 neonates of 100 mothers with COVID-19 found no infant was infected even though they were breastfeeding and rooming in (Dumitriu et al., 2020).

Milk samples usually show no evidence of COVID-19, but that is not always true. In a published case report, an uninfected premature baby who was accidentally fed expressed milk infected with COVID-19, did not become sick (Lugli et al., 2020). This case tells us that the virus *can* get into breastmilk. Even so, it did not make a vulnerable preterm baby sick.

## Hepatitis

### Hepatitis A

Hepatitis A or B can cause mothers to be easily fatigued, have abdominal pain, and lessen their appetite. Infection with hepatitis viruses often causes jaundice as well. The hepatitis virus is also present in bowel movements, which can infect others. Mothers may feel weak, which can make it difficult for them to care for their babies. The best course is for mothers to go to bed with their babies and breastfeed them in bed. While mothers are ill, they should not be responsible for routine care of their babies other than breastfeeding. Ideally, others can step in and help take care for both baby and mother.

Switching to formula does not keep babies from getting sick and probably makes them more vulnerable. If babies do get infected, continued breastfeeding decreases their risk of becoming ill. If they are ill, they usually do not become severely ill. After all, the virus infects via the intestinal tract, and the intestinal tract is where breastmilk immunity has its most profound protective effect. In any case, as with many viruses, hepatitis viruses are most infectious before the person realizes they are sick. In fact, as with many infections, infections with hepatitis viruses may be asymptomatic.

## Hepatitis B

Infection with hepatitis B is very similar to infection with hepatitis A, with the same symptoms: jaundice, fatigue, and abdominal pain. As with hepatitis A, not everyone who is infected develops the illness. However, unlike hepatitis A, about 10% to 15% become chronic carriers of the virus, which means that their bodily fluids may be infectious even if they never had symptoms of the disease.

Regarding symptomatic infection, by the time a mother develops symptoms, she may have already passed the virus to her baby, but not through her milk. There is no evidence that the virus enters the milk. Even when pregnant women are chronic carriers, breastfeeding is still recommended (Chen et al., 2013). However, most jurisdictions now recommend that babies born to mothers with hepatitis B (acute infection or chronic carrier) receive the hepatitis B vaccine *at birth* as well as be given hepatitis immune globulin *within 12 hours of birth.*

## Hepatitis C

The clinical picture of hepatitis C is like hepatitis A and B, though it is frequently milder and very often asymptomatic. As with hepatitis B, however, people can be chronic carriers. Chronic carriers can now be treated, but untreated carriers can develop cirrhosis of the liver. Most of medications used to treat chronic hepatitis C are molecules too large to get into milk. In addition, they are highly protein bound. (See Chapter 20 on medications and breastfeeding.)

There is no evidence *that breastfeeding transmit*s the infection if is quiescent and the nipples are not traumatized (Roberts & Young, 2002). However, mothers with hepatitis C infection need excellent lactation support, like all mothers in fact, to prevent trauma with possible bleeding from cracked nipples. The mother's blood may infect the baby.

### Herpes Viruses

At present, 8 or 9 different herpes viruses cause disease in humans and more will likely be discovered. Most infections with herpes viruses do not cause symptoms. However, herpes can cause sores on the skin, lips, mouth, genitals, and the conjunctiva of the eyes. Herpes viruses are also the cause chicken pox, infectious mononucleosis, and herpes zoster (shingles).

### Herpes Virus 1 and 2

These two viruses can cause infectious sores of the lips and mouth (herpes 1) and genitals (herpes 2, occasionally herpes 1). Most commonly, we see a breastfeeding toddler with herpes stomatitis, or ulcers in the mouth. These can be painful enough to prevent children from eating or drinking, though they *usually will* continue breastfeeding. In extreme cases, the child may even refuse to breastfeed or take breastmilk by cup. When they refuse *all liquids and food including breastfeeding, they may need to be admitted to the hospital for intravenous fluids to maintain hydration. If children continue breastfeeding, hospitalization is rarely needed as the* children will remain well hydrated and receive nutrients as well as immune factors that may shorten the course of their illness. Even if children are admitted to the hospital, they should return to breastfeed as soon as they are willing. Therefore, we should encourage mothers to stay with their children in the hospital as much as possible.

Sometimes, the breastfeeding mother develops sores on her nipples that can be very painful. As with the other infections, there is an incubation period of herpes virus. Usually, it is children who infect their mothers as the nipple would be an unusual location for the initial infection. Children may infect their mothers several days before they have sores. The following photo shows herpes virus infection of the nipples.

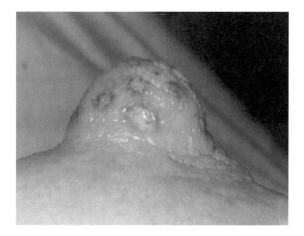

This photo shows the nipple of a mother whose toddler developed herpetic stomatitis (infection in the mouth) about 3 or 4 days before the mother developed these painful sores. She continued breastfeeding through the pain and in about 1 week, the sores were healing, and pain was gone.

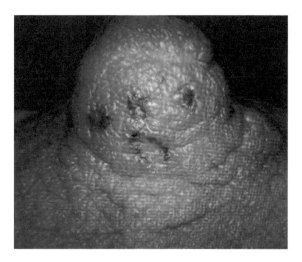

This photo is of the same mother's nipple 1 week later. Her pain has gone.

Mothers should continue breastfeeding if they can. If they cannot, hand expressing and feeding the expressed milk to the baby is better than pumping because hand expression does not put pressure on the nipples. If the child will take anything by mouth, the milk can be fed by cup or spoon, or mixed with solids.

Medications used to treat herpes virus 1 and 2, such as acyclovir and valacyclovir, do not require mothers to interrupt breastfeeding. Unfortunately, healthcare providers frequently tell mothers that they need to stop because of these medications. Interrupting breastfeeding for these medications is not good for either mother or child.

## Human Immunodeficiency Virus Infection (HIV)

The rule used to be that mothers with human immunodeficiency virus (HIV) could never breastfeed. This virus attacks and destroys the infected person's immune system and it can be transferred to the baby via breastmilk. Thus, until recently, breastfeeding was considered contraindicated where formula-feeding was considered safe and feasible.

However, the World Health Organization now considers breastfeeding safe and desirable *if* the pregnant woman as well as the baby immediately after birth are being treated with anti-retroviral medication (World Health Organization, 2010). The breastfeeding mother also should continue anti-viral medication. This recommendation is not always followed in Europe or North America, where artificial infant feeding is still considered "safer." However, we believe that mothers and babies should be treated and encouraged to breastfeed, given the risks of *not* breastfeeding. In Europe and the UK, there is a tendency to "allow" breastfeeding if the mother and baby are both treated and the mother desires ardently to breastfeed, but most health professionals do not actively encourage breastfeeding, and breastfeeding with HIV is not usual in these countries. In fact, health care professionals still worry that the baby is in danger if the mother breastfeeds.

On 30 November 2009, WHO released new recommendations on infant feeding by HIV-positive mothers, based on this new evidence.

For the first time, WHO is recommending that HIV-positive mothers or their infants take antiretroviral drugs throughout the period of breastfeeding and until the infant is 12 months old. This means that the child can benefit from breastfeeding with very little risk of becoming infected with HIV (p. 9).

## Human T Cell Leukemia Virus (HTLV)

There are two known forms of Human T cell leukemia virus (HTLV): 1 and 2. A study from Iran found that breastfeeding for less than 6 months did not increase risk of vertical transmission of HTLV, but breastfeeding for more than 6 months did (Boostani, Sadeghi, Sabouri, & Ghabeli-Juibary, 2018). The incidence may be lower than if the baby was not breastfed at all during the first 6 months. However, various studies do not agree. Most experts in the field still recommend no breastfeeding, although the following article suggests pasteurized breastmilk as an alternative to formula-feeding (Carneiro-Proietti et al., 2014).

## Influenza

Every year (except 2020), there is an epidemic of influenza. Generally, the Centers for Disease Control supports breastfeeding if mothers have the flu (Centers for Disease Control and Prevention, 2021). However, a couple of years ago, the CDC stated that mothers with suspected or proven influenza, should be separated from their babies and not even allowed to provide their milk (Centers for Disease Control and Prevention, 2020). We disagree with this and do not understand the evidence that supports such a statement. We strongly recommend that breastfeeding mothers be immunized against influenza.

## Lyme Disease

Lyme disease is known to be caused by at least four different bacteria. *Borrelia burgdorferi and Borrelia mayonii cause Lyme disease in North America, while Borrelia afzelii and Borrelia garinii are the leading causes* in Europe and Asia. Tick bites transmit the bacterium. The tick species that causes Lyme disease varies by geographical location.

Lyme disease can affect several systems of the body, including the skin, joints, heart, and central nervous system. Unilateral facial paralysis should make the physician consider the possibility of Lyme disease, even though it can be caused by other bacteria or other causes of inflammation. Some believe that a tick needs to be attached for at least 16 hours before the Lyme disease bacterium can infect the person who was bitten. However, transfer of the bacterium to animals, including humans, can take much less time and may occur soon after the tick attaches (Cook, 2015).

To date, living Lyme disease bacteria have *not* been found in breastmilk, though markers of the bacterium have been. However, even if the bacterium does pass into the milk, it's unlikely that it would have been able to bypass the immune-factor barriers, penetrate the intestinal wall, and get into the baby's bloodstream to cause infection.

The drug of choice for the treatment of Lyme disease, doxycycline, used to be considered contraindicated during breastfeeding because it could possibly damage babies' and young children's teeth. More recent evidence (Todd et al., 2015), however, has found this medication safe even when it's given directly to babies and children.

## Tuberculosis

Tuberculosis was always assumed to be transmissible through breastmilk. This may not be true; some articles state yes, others no. However, in order for the tuberculosis bacillus to enter the milk, it must be in the blood. Tuberculosis bacteria is not usually in the blood of an adult with TB. However, if tuberculosis is causing infection of the breast itself, transmission to the baby could occur. Nevertheless, if a mother has active tuberculosis, she should continue breastfeeding, and mother and baby both should both be treated.

## Non-Infectious Diseases

There is a wide range of inflammatory and autoimmune diseases, such as rheumatoid arthritis, lupus erythematosus, idiopathic thrombocytopenic purpura, autoimmune hemolytic anemia, autoimmune thyroiditis, which are caused by autoantibodies produced by the mother's body. Although men can get these diseases, they are much more common in women, frequently of childbearing age.

Many physicians believe that mothers with autoimmune disorders cannot breastfeed because the antibodies that cause these diseases enter the milk and cause autoimmunity in the baby. They completely misunderstand how breastmilk immunity works. There are several sorts of antibodies. The antibodies that cause autoimmune diseases differ from the antibodies in breastmilk that protect the baby from infection.

The antibodies (sIgA) in breastmilk require a special added protein chain to allow these antibodies to enter the milk. In addition, they have another chain that prevents the digestive enzymes in the stomach and gastrointestinal tract from destroying the antibodies. At least 90% of the antibodies found in breastmilk are sIgA. Therefore, antibodies causing mothers' disease do not enter the milk and make babies sick. Considering that breastfeeding helps babies develop a normal immune system and gut microbiome, we should encourage mothers to breastfeed exclusively for the recommended 6 months or so, and then continue for as long as she and the child desire.

## Conclusions

In most cases, mothers can and should continue to breastfeed with infectious diseases including HIV and COVID-19. Mothers with infections are almost universally contagious before they have symptoms, so babies have already been exposed to the illness before mothers show symptoms. Breastmilk works hand in hand with babies' own immune systems to protect them from illness or lessen symptoms if they do get sick. Mothers need practical help with day-to-day tasks while they are sick, so that they can rest and continue to breastfeed their babies.

## CHAPTER 20

# Maternal Medications and Breastfeeding

The breastfeeding question we receive most often is whether breast-feeding is safe while the mother is taking medications. Unfortunately, misinformation abounds. Mothers are frequently told they must interrupt breastfeeding if they take medication in order for the baby "to be safe." In the vast majority of situations, interruption of breastfeeding is unnecessary and potentially harmful if we follow the medical dictum, *primum non nocere* (Latin: "first, do no harm"). Fortunately, we have excellent resources on medications and breastfeeding and can offer guidance. In general, very few drugs are contraindicated during breastfeeding. There are some, which we will mention. However, we urge readers to *not* to assume a drug is contraindicated. Most commonly used drugs are not contraindicated in breastfeeding mothers.

## How Drugs Pass into Milk

A complete discussion of drugs and breastfeeding is not possible, but we can describe a few general rules. The vast majority of drugs are compatible with breastfeeding. If prescribing physicians are unsure, medication characteristics can help them figure out the answer.

### Medication Molecule Size

Many drugs have molecular weights greater than 600 to 800. If they do, the molecules are too large to pass into breastmilk. For example, monoclonal antibodies, some new cancer drugs, most of the drugs used to treat chronic hepatitis C are all large molecules. The molecular weight of any drug is easily found by searching "what is the molecular weight of (drug name)" online.

## Protein Binding

The percentage of drug bound to protein is another useful piece of information and is also readily available online. Protein binding results in a drug with a low molecular weight becoming a "large" drug, too large to get into milk. If a drug is 98% bound to protein (not unusual), then only 2% of the drug can enter the milk.

## Volume of Distribution

The volume of distribution of a drug essentially gives an indication of whether a drug is mostly in the blood or distributed elsewhere in the body. The volume of distribution is also relatively easy to find online though the units that measure volume of distribution seem to change, making things more complicated. It may be necessary to search for, "What is the volume of distribution of..." A large volume of distribution means that most of the drug is not in the blood (having been dispersed to other parts of the body, such as the brain). Antidepressants are a good example of medications that distribute to the brain as they need to be there to do their job. For example, sertraline (Zoloft), an SSRI antidepressant, has a volume of distribution of 20 litres/kg. This is a very large volume of distribution.

These three characteristics of medications provide enough information for the prescribing physician to know whether that medication enters the milk in significant amounts. It also helps to know if that a drug is poorly absorbed from the baby's intestinal tract. A medication that babies do not absorb is unlikely to negatively affect them.

# Non-Useful Sources

## Package Inserts

Information in package inserts almost always says something like, "If you are breastfeeding, consult your doctor about the advisability of continuing breastfeeding while on this medication." Pharmaceutical companies put the onus on doctors. Doctors are usually not knowledgeable enough about drugs and breastfeeding to make these kinds of decisions and feel out of their depth in advising breastfeeding mothers. Or they frequently respond, "No, you cannot continue breastfeeding." Just to be "safe." It is not fair to put this on doctors. Most have learned nothing about breastfeeding during their training or after. Remember that many doctors may have children who were not breastfed. (If you don't think that is not a consideration, you are wrong.)

## Most Doctors

Many doctors, including many pediatricians, do not know this, the topic of this entire book.

## Many Pharmacists

Unfortunately, on the topic of medications and *breastfeeding,* many pharmacists are no more knowledgeable than most doctors.

## Online Information

There are many unreliable sources online. With regard to breastfeeding, it is best to be cautious about online information. Fortunately, there are some good sources. Two of the best include the Infant Risk Center and the U.S. National Institute of Health's LactMed database.

### The Mother's Best Friend, or Her Cousin, or the Baby's Grandmother

Friends and family are often cautious and may advise weaning when it is not necessary.

## There Are Risks Associated with Not Breastfeeding

Some people only consider the risks of breastfeeding while on medications, but that equation is incomplete. That consideration must be balanced with the risks of *not* breastfeeding. That risk usually far exceeds the risk of any potential exposure to medications via milk. So, what are the risks of not breastfeeding? A meta-analysis in the journal *Lancet* (Victora et al., 2016) concluded that breastfeeding gives,

> … protection against child infections and malocclusion, increases in intelligence, and probable reductions in overweight and diabetes. We did not find associations with allergic disorders such as asthma or with blood pressure or cholesterol, and we noted an increase in tooth decay with longer periods of breastfeeding. For nursing women, breastfeeding gave protection against breast cancer, and it improved birth spacing, and it might also protect against ovarian cancer and type 2 diabetes (p. 475).

With regard to the above study by Victora et al. (2016), we do not agree with the increase in tooth decay with longer periods of breastfeeding. It just does not make sense. This notion is based on the definite association of bottle-feeding formula (or even, perhaps, breastmilk in a bottle). Breastfeeding at night differs from babies fed formula, sugar water, or even breastmilk in a propped bottle. Breastfeeding involves the nipple far back in the baby's mouth. Unlike with the propped bottle, where the milk bathes the mouth and teeth for long periods, a baby breastfeeding at night swallows the milk immediately and the teeth are not bathed with milk.

Some of the connections between breastfeeding and later disease development are difficult to determine as there are many factors that contribute to child and adult health including heredity (W. Oddy, 2017). In addition, with regard to formula, there are thorny questions of how much is too much. For example, what if the baby is mostly breastfeeding, but gets a bottle of formula from time to time? Or what if the baby received a few bottles of formula in hospital but then was exclusively breastfed to 6 months and continued breastfeeding until 2 years of age? Should such babies be eliminated from the study? Very few babies, unfortunately, would be available to study if the criteria were that they have never had formula.

The bottom line is this: breastfeeding is the *biological norm* and there is evidence that breastfeeding lowers the risk of many diseases. If that is true, the converse is also true: formula increases the risk of disease. At times, feeding a baby formula may be unavoidable. However, in almost all cases, the "use formula just to be safe" argument does not stand up.

## Does Interrupting Breastfeeding Qualify as Non Nocere (Do No Harm)?

In the vast majority of cases, *absolutely not*. Interrupting breastfeeding, even for a few days, may lead to breast refusal. Bottle-feeding and breast-feeding are not interchangeable. Introducing bottles, even for a short time, can mean the end of breastfeeding. While it is true that many babies do go back and forth, some babies cannot manage that transition. Is it worth risking possible breastfeeding cessation when it is likely not necessary? There's a lot at stake and it is worth doing some homework before deciding.

## Medications that Never Enter Milk

Medications that are large molecules will not get into milk and will there-fore not negatively affect the baby or toddler. Below is a listing of some of the more common classes of medications with large molecules.

### Monoclonal Antibodies

Monoclonal antibodies are now being used to treat many diseases including COVID-19; cancer, including leukemia and lymphoma; autoimmune disorders, such as rheumatoid arthritis, ulcerative colitis, Crohn's disease, psoriasis, severe asthma, and kidney rejection after transplantation. Perhaps in the near future, there will be a monoclonal antibody for all diseases humans are susceptible to.

Monoclonal antibodies pose no risk to the baby. The molecules are huge—too large to get into milk. Infliximab, one of the earliest of the monoclonal antibodies available for use, has a molecular weight of 144,000: at least 185 times too large to get into the milk. Most monoclonal antibodies have similar molecular weights.

These medications are antibodies and antibodies are proteins. Even if they entered the milk, which they do not, the stomach acid and enzymes in the baby's stomach would destroy them. But they do not get into the milk. Mothers have antibodies in their milk to help protect the baby from infection (secretory IgA) and these *do* get into the milk. However, the breastmilk antibodies mothers make have an added chain, which other proteins/antibodies do not. That extra chain allows secretory IgA to enter the milk. Another chain protects them from being destroyed in the babies' stomachs. Monoclonal antibodies do not have this chain either.

## Botox

Botulinum toxin (Botox) does not get into the milk because it stays where it is injected. If it did not stay where injected, if it entered the mother's blood, it could kill her. Drugs that do not get into the mother's blood cannot get into milk. But even if it did enter the blood (it does not), Botox is too large a molecule to get into the milk. Believe it or not, Botox and breastfeeding is one of the most frequent questions we receive. Our advice? Do not interrupt breastfeeding!

## Heparin

Even lower molecular weight heparin cannot get into the milk because the molecule is too large. Even if it did, the baby's stomach would destroy it.

## Fertility Drugs

Most hormones, such as luteinizing hormone and follicle stimulating hormone, frequently used in fertility treatments are too big to get into the milk.

## Insulin and Newer Drugs for Diabetes

Insulin has a molecular weight of almost 6000, too large to get into the milk. Glucagon-like peptide-1 receptor agonists (GLP-1), such as liraglutide, are relatively new treatments for type 2 diabetes. Liraglutide and the other drugs of the family are also huge molecules with a molar mass, in the case of liraglutide, of 3,751,262 g/mol. Thus, they will not enter the milk.

## CT Scans or MRIs

Sometimes, mothers are told to stop breastfeeding so that they can have a CT scan or MRI. Mothers are told to interrupt breastfeeding for 24 to 48 hours so they can have these scans. There is no need to interrupt breast-feeding at all, not even for a minute. See this statement from the American College of Radiologists (2021) which says that there is no need to interrupt breastfeeding for the contrast used in these tests. The statement does muddy the waters by saying "if the mother is concerned, she can interrupt breast-feeding for 24 hours." Well, Dr. Radiologist, if you answered instead that "there is no concern," as recommended by your own College, the mother would not be concerned, would she?

## Cancer Medications

Cisplatin, used to treat some types of cancer, was long considered incom-patible with breastfeeding, but now is considered to be compatible. It has >90% protein binding and is not absorbed from the intestinal tract. Both characteristics suggest that cisplatin is safe for the breastfeeding baby when the mother takes it. The small amount in the milk is diluted in intestinal fluid and ends up in the baby's bowel movements. Significant contact with the mucosa of the baby's intestinal tract, causing harm to the mucosal cells, is very unlikely. Though cisplatin is sometimes used with other drugs that may contraindicate breastfeeding, often it is the only drug the mother receives.

Two relatively new anti-cancer drugs, docetaxel (molecular weight of: 808 g/mol; oral absorption: 0; protein binding >98%) and paclitaxel (molecular weight: 853.918 g/mol; Oral absorption 6.5%; protein binding

89-98%) are extremely unlikely to enter the milk. The molecular weights are borderline but the protein binding and poor absorption from the gut make any significant exposure of the baby to these drugs extremely unlikely.

## Some Antibiotics Enter Milk but Babies Do Not Absorb Them

Aminoglycoside antibiotics are a family of antibiotics that includes gentamicin, tobramycin, and vancomycin. The intestinal tract does not absorb these antibiotics. Mothers (and any patient) usually receive these drugs by injection. They enter into milk but are *not* absorbed from the baby's intestinal tract. They leave babies' bodies in their bowel movements. Yes, these antibiotics will likely change the microbiome of the intestinal tract, but then, so will taking babies off the breast and feeding them formula. If mothers continue breastfeeding, and breast-feeding exclusively, presumably, perhaps, the microbiome will change back to what it was before the mother took the antibiotics.

Vancomycin is sometimes given orally to patients for intestinal infections such as *C. difficile*, a serious, occasionally fatal, infection of the intestinal tract. Vancomycin cannot get into milk because it is not absorbed from the mother's intestinal tract. Interestingly, gentamicin is still used to treat possible sepsis in premature babies. This was true in 1980 and is still true today.

Doxycycline is an antibiotic that used to be contraindicated for breastfeeding, but no longer is. It is used for diseases such as malaria, Rocky Mountain spotted fever, and Lyme disease. The concern was that it could cause permanent staining and weakness of children's teeth, like tetracycline. Studies of children being treated for malaria with doxycycline, however, have found no significant changes in their teeth (Gaillard, Briolant, Madamet, & Pradines, 2017). Children are treated with it directly, so it is also considered safe for breastfeeding.

# Radioactive Iodine is Contraindicated

## Thyroid Cancer

Mothers on radioactive iodine, used to treat thyroid cancer, need to interrupt breastfeeding for at least a month as there is significant excretion of radioactivity into breastmilk. Furthermore, mothers treated with radioactive iodine should not have any close physical contact with their babies or other people for at least a week, as radioactivity comes out in the mother's sweat and other secretions. Most babies will not take the breast after a month off the breast, but some will go right back to it. Mothers can save their expressed milk in a safe place and use it after about 6 weeks. It is no longer radioactive after 5 half-lives (the half-life of radioactive iodine 131 is 8 days, so 5 times the half-life is 40 days). Babies over 6 months of age can be fed food from a spoon, or can eat with their hands, and drink liquids from an open cup. Babies who do not receive bottles or pacifiers would be more likely to take the breast again after about 5 weeks, though they may not.

A complicating factor is that endocrinologists recommend that mothers dry up their milk (by not feeding or pumping) before the mother receives the radioactive iodine. The reason is that breast cells are very active metabolically, and thus may take up more radiation, with the possible long-term negative effects, including increased risk of breast cancer. This approach is based on the belief that breastfeeding can be stopped but making blood cells cannot. In other words, giving radioactive iodine may also slightly increase the risk of the patient developing leukemia.

For this reason, we recommend that radioactive iodine not be given unless there is evidence of cancer spreading to the lymph nodes, for example, or a more aggressive type of cancer. Often, cancer of the thyroid is limited to the thyroid, and in young women, cancer tends to be the less aggressive type: papillary carcinoma. Therefore, surgery alone, without radioactive iodine and close follow-up may be a better option for breastfeeding mothers. The mother could go back to breastfeeding immediately after the surgery, as neither the anesthetic given during surgery, nor the drugs for pain after, require the mother not to breastfeed.

Endocrinologists also will not recommend pumping to maintain the milk supply after the radioactive iodine treatment. After radioactive iodine is given, the patient is told to get rid of the radioactive iodine as quickly as possible by drinking lots of liquids (radioactivity in urine), eating high-fiber foods (radioactivity in bowel movements), and take frequent showers to wash off sweat which also contains radioactive iodine. So why not use frequent pumping to get it out of the body? (The radioactivity in any remaining thyroid tissue will stay attached there.) We think mothers should have all this information and be part of the decision-making process.

## Graves' Disease

When treating Graves' Disease (hyperthyroidism), many endocrinologists recommend radioactive iodine, believing, perhaps, that it is simpler and avoids surgery. Simpler, perhaps, for the treating physician. However, it also requires isolation until the person is no longer a radiation hazard to others, as with thyroid cancer, with careful discarding of urine and bowel movements as well careful handling of clothing and bedding, so maybe it is not *that* simple. It has the significant advantage of not being painful. Although the dose of radiation for Graves' disease is much smaller than it is for thyroid cancer, it still requires that mothers interrupt breastfeeding for at least a month.

On the other hand, surgery does not require a significant separation of mother and baby (the drugs used for general anesthetic and after the surgery, including narcotics, do *not* require interruption of breastfeeding). In true Baby-Friendly hospitals, the breastfeeding baby would be admitted with the mother so breastfeeding can continue.

We think that surgery is the better alternative from the perspective of continued breastfeeding compared to radioactive iodine. Naturally, in our baby-unfriendly hospitals, mothers and babies may be separated for a day or two or more. At the very least, we hope that these baby-unfriendly hospitals would allow the baby to visit frequently (and breastfeed) until mothers can be discharged.

## Hormonal Contraception

People often ask whether hormonal contraception is compatible with breastfeeding. Birth control pills and IUDs that release progesterone are the most commonly prescribed female hormones. Unfortunately, they are a problem. In some breastfeeding mothers, it is so obvious. The mother starts the pill or has the IUD with progesterone inserted. Within a week or two, the baby starts fussing and pulling at the breast. It is clear to anyone who listens that something is affecting the baby's satisfaction and drinking at the breast.

The cervical ring, which releases estrogen into the mother's blood stream, comes with a warning that it may cause breast tenderness and swelling. Perhaps that is just "covering the pharmaceutical company's risk" but it strongly suggests that estrogen enters the mother's bloodstream, and it affects her. There is no question that estrogen decreases mothers' milk supply and the flow of milk to the baby.

Kapp and Curtis (2010) concluded that progestin-only pills or IUDs do not affect breastmilk production or infant growth. Our experience suggests otherwise. Furthermore, we believe that it is too risky for the mother's milk supply to prescribe any female hormones during lactation (except for trans women who should continue *physiological* doses of estrogen and progesterone). There are multiple methods of birth control that do not require female hormones. The pill is very easy for the physician to prescribe and seems easy for mothers. An option might be the copper IUD, which does not release hormones.

## Lactation Amenorrhea Method (LAM)

Health professionals in affluent countries rarely mention the lactation amenorrhea method (LAM), which is very effective for at least 6 months, if followed as recommended. That means exclusive breastfeeding with no schedule, feedings around the clock, no artificial nipples such as pacifiers (Tiwari, Khanam, & Savarna, 2018). Even after 6 months it gives decreasing, but still significant protection.

If mothers breastfeed into the second year of life, fertility usually returns between 14 and 17 months after birth. It is true that many breastfeeding mothers could not use this method because their baby is using a pacifier or receiving bottles.

Breastfeeding mothers can also use the cervical mucus method of predicting with accuracy which days of their cycle they are likely to be fertile, thus combining breastfeeding with knowledge of when the mother becomes fertile to prevent pregnancy (Bigelow et al., 2004). This is another useful bit of information that most couples are not aware of.

Bigelow and colleagues (2004) describe the increased chance of pregnancy on the days when the cervical mucus is "transparent, like raw egg white, stretchy/elastic, liquid, watery, or reddish." This method is not known to most health professionals, it seems. Or they view it, like anything that does not come out of medication factories, as untrustworthy. For the days when the mother is likely to become pregnant, the couple can abstain, use a condom, or enjoy sex without penetration.

## Fertility Treatments

Breastfeeding women typically experience lactational amenorrhea after birth for various length of time. This is normal and there is no *definite* fixed time for women's menstrual cycle to return if she is breastfeeding exclusively and has no problems. Even during the period of lactational amenorrhea, mothers can observe the possible return of her menstrual cycle and ovulation.

Some women may need fertility treatment. In these situations, breastfeeding women are often told that the medication is incompatible with continued breastfeeding and to get treatment, they must first stop breastfeeding. Furthermore, if women wish to become pregnant, they are often told that stopping breastfeeding is a condition for them to receive treatment because breastfeeding decreases their chances of becoming and staying pregnant. However, once the women's cycle returns, after the first three postpartum cycles, breastfeeding no longer affects the woman's fertility and pregnancy is possible.

Letrozole used off-label and clomiphene are both said to be contraindicated during breastfeeding. Fertility clinics usually tell women to stop breastfeeding in case they need to take these medications. Treating the mother with progesterone, as discussed in the section on birth control, will likely decrease the milk supply. The decrease in milk supply caused by progesterone would probably ensure that very little of either the clomiphene or letrozole would get to the child as there would be very little breastmilk for the child to drink.

On the other hand, taking progesterone or HCG injections are no problem in breastfeeding women. The only consideration is that both will likely decrease the mother's milk supply and her child may react negatively to the decrease. If the mother gets pregnant, her milk supply will also decrease. Furthermore, injections of luteinizing hormone (LH) and follicle stimulating hormone (FSH) are used to induce ovulation and apparently work well, but perhaps not as well as letrozole and clomiphene. Neither LH nor FSH are contraindicated during breastfeeding though they may decrease milk supply.

## Ectopic Pregnancy

Methotrexate is frequently used when mothers have an ectopic pregnancy and mothers are told to stop breastfeeding for 1 or 2 days. We recently received an email where the mother was never told how long to take the medication and when she could start breastfeeding again. The baby had been off the breast for a week already. The mother probably didn't even need to stop while taking this medication.

## Conclusion

Mothers are frequently told to stop breastfeeding when prescribed medications. Practitioners often suggest formula, "just to be safe." Unfortunately, telling mothers to stop breastfeeding while on medication is, in most cases, completely unnecessary. And stopping breastfeeding is not necessarily "safe," not for the mother or the baby. Most medications are compatible with breastfeeding. The molecular weight and percentage of protein binding are good indicators of whether the medication will pass into the milk in any significant amounts or not. If the molecules are large, babies' exposure is minimal. In addition, the risk associated with medications in breastmilk must be balanced with the risks of formula use. In almost all cases, formula poses a greater risk for the baby than breastmilk and medication.

# INFANCY AND BEYOND

# CHAPTER 21

# Starting the Baby on Food

When babies are about 4 months old, many parents will notice that babies become interested in what their parents are eating. The baby will watch as food goes from their parents' plates to their mouths. By *approximately* 6 months of age, most babies will try to grab food, put it into their mouths, and eat. With their actions, they tell parents that, "I am ready to eat food. I want that chicken leg!" The baby in the photo below is not quite 6 months of age but is clearly interested in food.

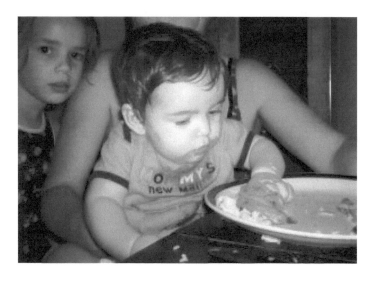

I (JN) remember when our firstborn was 6 months old and ate his first bit of food. I had just cut up some steak for his mother. He grabbed a piece, shoved it in his mouth, and chewed on it for at least 15 minutes, eventually spitting it out. (I do not remember if he had any teeth, but I think he did.)

We got the message. From then on, he ate whatever he wanted from our plates, and he never had difficulty eating.

Well, okay, at some point, we did try to feed him infant cereal. After all, I was about to start my residency in pediatrics, and I knew the "rules." He allowed us to put the cereal in his mouth and promptly spat it out. We got *that* message too, and never offered him cereal again. We dare anyone reading this to eat infant cereal and "love it."

The point is that babies want the same food as the rest of the family. They are social beings and want to participate in the same activities as their parents and siblings. Babies are very different at 6 months than they were at 2 or 4 months. They mimic the adults' behavior. Furthermore, babies can and should be eating without someone spooning food into their mouths. They can pick up the food and eat it without help. It can be messy, but if the parents don't like messes, it is time to get over that.

## Can Babies Eat Food Before 6 Months?

Some babies seem eager to start solids a little earlier than 6 months of age. Must parents wait until the magical 6 months? Not necessarily. We both agree with the World Health Organization's recommended 6 months of exclusive breastfeeding, but that is a public health statement. Not all babies follow the "rule" and individual situations may vary. Thus, if a baby wants to start, say, 1 week early, that's reasonable. We often receive emails where mothers (or others) are concerned about an almost 6-month-old baby's weight gain. When we recommend starting the baby on food, a common reply is, "But he won't be 6 months until next week." Seriously? We also recommend increasing breastmilk intake, but in this situation, starting food 1 week early makes sense, no? What about 2 weeks early? In our view, it's better to add food 2 weeks "early," than formula, which usually implies starting bottles that would undermine breastfeeding.

What sort of food should babies be eating at the age of 6 months? Essentially whatever the parents are eating, assuming they are eating nutritious food themselves. Babies do not need special foods, purees, or infant cereal. They don't need to avoid allergenic foods. If the parents or siblings are not eating nutritious food, it might be time to change their eating habits. Babies can also start drinking water from an open cup. They don't need sippy cups, which are essentially modified bottles. We have photos of young babies drinking from wine or shot glasses.

## What about Choking?

In the 21st century, we assume that starting babies on regular food is dangerous. True, babies can choke on food, but so can adults. With reasonable care, there is no reason that this should occur in a 6-month-old baby any more than in an adult, and that special precautions are necessary.

However, babies should not be given anything round and slippery. (The Hospital for Sick Children in Toronto once displayed foods removed from young children's lungs including popcorn and peanuts.) However, Health Canada's suggestion to cut blueberries in half makes us wonder if anyone would ever do that. Blueberries are hardly essential foods and parents can introduce them into the child's diet when the child is older. In any case, is it less likely a baby would choke on half a blueberry than a whole blueberry? Just asking!

As long as parents are nearby, babies can safely eat some surprising things. In the first photo, an 8-month-old baby is chewing on a chicken bone. Is that safe? Yes, babies are unlikely to choke on something this big and it probably feels pretty good if they are cutting teeth.

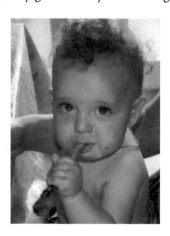

Babies can also eat meat if their parents are right there, and the piece is big enough for them to hold. It wouldn't be safe to leave them unsupervised, but that's true for any type of food. Babies tend to gnaw on rather than swallow meat. They do manage to suck the nutrients and flavor from it, which they seem to enjoy. The baby is this picture is about 8 months old.

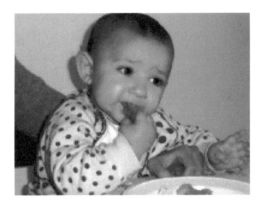

In this lovely photo, baby and mother are eating the same food.

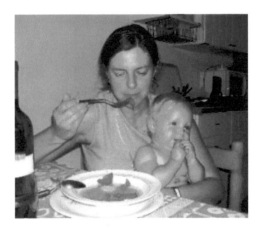

Why do babies like eating with their parents? Because eating is social. "Give us this day our daily bread," with the family around the table is no longer the norm, it seems. But maybe, if we reinforce the social nature of meals by letting babies and children eat the same foods as the rest of the family. Maybe families eating together can once again be the norm.

## What about Breastfeeding?

Once a baby is 6 months old, we tend to focus on food ("real" food as grandparents often call it) and pay less attention to breastfeeding. Many believe that breastmilk no longer contains nutrients that babies need to stay healthy and grow. Does that make sense? If breastfeeding is all babies need at 5 months, how did it become devoid of nutrients at 6 months? It isn't. Breastfeeding still provides for most of babies' nutritional needs even after they start eating food. Many babies could continue to gain weight well *on breastfeeding alone* for several months longer than the first 6 months (though they might require iron supplements). We do not recommend this, but there *might* be circumstances that warrant it.

Food is not a substitute for breastfeeding and breastfeeding is not a supplement to food. Breastfeeding is still the main food, something that many health professionals do not understand or appreciate. If breastfeeding problems appear past 6 months, they do not mean that the baby is "self-weaning." Babies do not self-wean before the age of 2.5 or 3 years of age. The time between 6 months and 2 years gives babies time to learn to eat all the same food adults eat.

## Food Products That Breastfed Babies Do Not Need

Starting solids refers to adding family foods to breastfeeding. Unfortunately, companies see this transition as yet another opportunity to sell things to parents that neither they nor their babies need; the infant/child feeding market brings in billions each year. If mothers are breastfeeding, none of these products are necessary.

### Infant Formula

We, obviously, do not agree with routine introduction of formula. The breastfeeding couple is a unit. They belong together and should not be separated, even by a bottle, unless necessary. Even if mothers are hospitalized or need medication, breastfeeding families can find a way to make this work. Early breastfeeding support prevents the need for infant formula. Of course, if a mother requires hospitalization, it is best the baby be admitted with the mother, so that breastfeeding is continued. It does a lot of good for the baby and usually also a lot of good for a sick mother.

Unfortunately, many healthcare professionals encourage parents to introduce bottles and formula even if breastfeeding is going well. This is completely unnecessary. They often say, "in case you are separated from your baby, the baby will have something to drink." Or they say, "babies need something in their bodies besides breastmilk so that the 'shock' of food after 6 months won't be too great." We have heard this nonsense one more than once. The other classic is, "give your partner a chance to feed the baby so that they won't feel left out." Babies obviously do not need to be held, played with, talked to, bathed, have their diapers changed, or sung to. There is only feeding; that is all that matters. ("She gets all the fun with the baby, and I get the diaper changes.") Interestingly, when it comes to feeding the baby "real" food after 6 months, many (not all) such partners will pass on that after the initial excitement.

## Follow-On or Toddler Formula

Toddler formulas are pure marketing hype and completely unnecessary. They are touted as a way of maintaining good nutrition for the baby/toddler until 3- or even 5 years of age but cost four times as much as ordinary cows' milk. The American Academy of Pediatrics, the Academy of Nutrition and Dietetics, the American Academy of Pediatric Dentistry, and the American Heart Association, in a 2019 consensus statement, also do not recommend toddler formulas (Lott, Callahan, Welker Duffy, Story, & Daniels, 2019). *The Atlantic* magazine also identified them as dangerous (Khazan, 2020). Even if a baby never breastfed, a regular diet of a wide variety of foods is all that is necessary for adequate nutrition. For toddlers, infant formula, or even cows' milk, are not necessary for good nutrition.

This is not to say that breastfeeding is no longer necessary or important. Breastfeeding is still very important for toddlers. It's not only for the breastmilk, but the relationship. And yes, they still get the same immune protection for as long as they breastfeed.

### Commercial Infant Cereals

These cereals are bland, expensive, and completely unnecessary. Indeed, the nutritional value of most commercial cereals is rather lacking. We think they are tasteless and believe most adults would agree. We wonder whether the mania for fast foods, which are high in fat and salt, could partially be a response to babies eating tasteless, manufactured first foods in infancy. We have no proof for this statement, of course. It's just a hypothesis.

Commercial infant cereals also have an interesting history, which explains why so many doctors think they are necessary. In 1930, three pediatricians working at the Hospital for Sick Children in Toronto, invented a first food for infants called Pablum, which was marketed widely. They invented this food to prevent nutritional deficiencies in young babies. This was at the beginning of the Great Depression when many families were living in poverty. It was also a time when many families did not know what babies should be eating, Pablum was a reliable way to ensure that babies got what they needed. Not true, but it was good marketing.

Unfortunately, the hospital sold the rights to Pablum to Mead Johnson, a major formula manufacturer. The Hospital for Sick Children, where the three pediatricians worked, now had a commercial reason for promoting the sale of Pablum. They received royalties from Pablum sales, a mutually beneficial relationship that ended only in 2005. This raises serious questions about the profitable relationship between an infant formula company and a major North American pediatric teaching hospital. As medical students and postgraduate doctors training at the Hospital for Sick Children we were taught to start the baby on Pablum as a first food, not "infant cereal," but "Pablum," a trade name.

Thus, in 2021, many family doctors and pediatricians throughout Canada, and the Centers for Disease Control in the U.S., recommend infant cereal as the first food. In Canada, the first food recommendation always seems to be "Pablum." In March 2021, a mother at our clinic told us that her *young* pediatrician said to add infant cereal to the baby's bottle; the baby was 2 months old. The mind boggles! What are pediatricians learning in their training?

### Introducing Gluten

Some earlier studies suggested that parents should introduce gluten into babies' diets early, in order to prevent celiac disease. Cereal makers used this research to justify their products. However, an excellent recent study concluded that "the time to first introduction to gluten introduction was not an independent risk factor for developing CD (celiac disease)" (Aronsson et al., 2015). In any case, there is no need for infant cereals to expose the baby to gluten (see photo). *This baby is being exposed to gluten in a tastier manner than with infant cereal.*

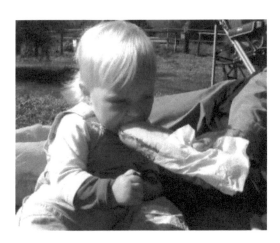

### Added Iron

Iron is the only ingredient added to commercial cereals thought to be of possible value after 6 months of age. In truth, added iron serves only to market the product. Unfortunately, added iron is constipating and poorly absorbed. Most of it ends up in the baby's diaper.

Is it necessary for babies to eat foods *fortified* with iron? Iron is a nutrient that many nutritionists misunderstood with regard to breast-milk and breastfeeding. Nutrition researchers took a wrong turn when they determined that the concentration of iron in breastmilk is "too low." Formula companies responded to that discovery by adding it to their products. What researchers did not understand was that exclusively breastfed, thriving babies are the *physiological norm*. If iron is "low" in breastmilk, there must be a reason. We now know that lower iron levels help prevent infection when exclusively breastfed babies start food (Quinn, 2014). The author postulates that high levels of iron encourage the growth of pathogenic bacteria because they need iron to multiply. Once babies are 6 months old and eating food and more iron, their immunity has developed, along with the immunity provided by breastfeeding, to the point where they can usually fight off infections.

## Food Pouches

The food industry never misses a chance to make money on unnecessary products. They now have pureed food in pouches for young babies. With food pouches, babies can suck on the pouch "nipple" and feed themselves any time they want to eat, even when being pushed along in a stroller or sitting in the parent's backpack. The entire notion of eating together has been lost with these food pouches. Even at the dinner table, these pouches mean different food for the baby, partly overcome, perhaps, by the absurd image of having the rest of the children eating from these pouches at the dinner table.

Although pouches may seem inexpensive, they are not compared to eating food from family plates. Food pouches also contradict Health Canada's recommendation that babies over 6 months of age should not eat purees, but rather family foods (Health Canada, Canadian Paediatric Society, Dietitians of Canada, & Breastfeeding Committee for Canada, 2014). Think about all these unrecyclable containers. Who is paying for them? Not the companies who make them.

That is not the only problem. Food pouches are often loaded with sugar, with some containing as much as than 6 Tablespoons (90 grams) per serving according to an article in the *Washington Post* (Reiley, 2019). Naturally, the sweetness of the product tempts babies, who are not necessarily hungry. Interesting how things turn around. As medical students, we were taught that eating a lot of sugar does not cause diabetes. Now we know that sugar contributes to childhood and adult overweight and obesity and thus, indirectly, to type 2 diabetes. Furthermore, food pouches are just a different sort of bottle. Some lactation consultants have noticed that many babies start to have difficulty with breastfeeding when they spend time "eating" (sucking) from food pouches, with corresponding late onset decreasing milk supply.

### Slow Down, You Move Too Fast

Breastfeeding is a marvelous way to slow down in this hectic world. If breastfeeding mothers are out with their babies and the babies are hungry, they can find a bench to sit on, stop, and breastfeed their children. On the other hand, the food pouch allows babies to eat and mothers to get things done on the run. Many might view this as a good thing, but something important is lost.

## When Older Babies Stop Gaining Weight—Ketosis

In other cases, when the mother's milk supply has decreased significantly, the baby may stay on the breast or have a pacifier in his mouth much of the day. The baby on the breast much of the day without gaining weight is often interpreted by those who do not know how to tell whether the baby is drinking or not drinking at the breast, as: "there is no nutritional value to breastmilk after a certain age" often stated as after 6 months or 1 year of age.

The real problem is not that there is no nutritional value in the breast-milk in this situation, but rather that the baby is not getting much milk from the breast. What so many health professionals do not understand is that a baby is not drinking milk simply because the baby is latched on to the breast and making sucking motions with his mouth.

And yet, it seems to make no sense that a baby not receiving enough milk to gain weight would refuse to eat solids. This is taken as proof positive by many pediatricians and nutritionists that there "is nothing in breastmilk after the first few months." But they can only say this because they do not watch the baby on the breast, and even if they did, they would not know what to watch for.

On the other hand, the mother is told that the baby is using too much energy sucking all day long and using up the calories he gets from the breast. But this too is a misconception, based on the notion that babies "transfer milk." Babies don't transfer milk, mothers do. Babies, of course, do their part in the breastfeeding process, their sucking stimulates the milk to flow from the breast. The baby is not a passive vessel, after all.

But why would the baby refuse solids if he's gaining little or no weight? It is true that the baby is not getting a lot of nutrients and calories, not because there is nothing in breastmilk after the first few months but rather because the baby is not getting much milk at all, period. This makes the baby *ketotic*, just like dieters on some fad diets. The purpose of which is to induce ketosis in the dieter. When you are ketotic, you lose your appetite. Thus, the baby has no interest in eating solids but continues on the breast because he gets comfort and security from it, another concept many health professionals still do not understand.

The other illogical deduction often made in such situations is that the baby is on the breast all the time, and thus filling up with so much breastmilk that he's not hungry. But if that were the case, the baby would be gaining weight just fine because there are a lot of calories and nutrients in breastmilk, enough to make a baby double his birthweight after 3 to 4 months of breastfeeding exclusively. A baby is not getting milk from the breast just because he is latched on and making sucking motions.

## Conclusion

Eating is a social event that usually involves the whole family interacting. When babies are ready for solids, they should eat family foods. With reasonable precautions, such as always having someone with the baby, they can enjoy most foods, but some foods are well-known choking hazards and should not be given to young babies.

# CHAPTER 22

# Infant Sleep and Sleep Training

**TO SLEEP, PERCHANCE TO DREAM**
**(from Hamlet's most famous soliloquy)**

Sleep is important and something families worry about a lot. New parents receive more advice about sleep than anything else, even more, if possible, than about what to feed the baby. Unfortunately, much of the advice that parents receive about sleep is inappropriate for breastfeeding mothers and their babies because its principles are based on formula-feeding.

We now know that feeding method is intrinsically related to infant sleep. Advice based on formula-feeding mothers' experience does not work for those who are breastfeeding. It's not only ineffective, but it can cause harm. For example, some psychologists and psychiatrists in our area recommend that mothers at risk for postpartum depression not breastfeed their babies at night. The idea is that someone else can feed the baby so that mothers can sleep through the night. They recommend this regimen to prevent postpartum depression and suggest that mothers start it from the very first days after birth.

This is not good advice. Indeed, we find this idea outrageous and following it will cause breastfeeding to fail. Within a short period, it will cause problems such as decreased milk supply and possible complete breast refusal. These problems will not help mothers at risk for postpartum depression who will see breastfeeding failure, which is almost guaranteed with this advice, as a personal failure, which increases their risk of depression (Borra et al., 2015).

We saw the result of such advice recently in the mother a 4-month-old baby. From the beginning, the parents were advised not to breastfeed at night. The baby received pumped milk or formula by bottle so that the mother could sleep 6 hours straight. The result? The mother's milk supply decreased. The baby continued to latch on to the breast for awhile, but "needed" bottles even during the day. Now, at the visit at 4 months, he refuses the breast completely. The mother is terribly stressed by this and is ready to do anything to relactate (See Chapter 17). Did her psychiatrist do her and her baby a favor?

## What is Normal Infant Sleep?

There are many myths about infant sleep. In fact, people have been "losing sleep" because of what they think about sleep. Most infant-sleep myths surfaced in the past 100 years, starting with erroneous assumption that formula-fed babies are the "model" for baby behavior. Health professionals have forgotten how babies sleep and what is normal. Many believe that there is only one correct way for babies (and adults) to sleep: 8 hours of uninterrupted sleep. Anyone who does not sleep that way is diagnosed with a "sleep problem." Interesting, this is a fairly new belief. Until recently, sleeping 8 consecutive hours was not considered normal even for adults (Hegarty, 2012). References from Homer's time (not Homer Simpson, Homer the Greek poet) to the 17th century describe a first sleep that began about two hours after dusk, followed by waking period of one or two hours, and then a second sleep.

The myths about sleep problems are particularly pernicious when it comes to infant sleep. Many believe that they can "turn babies off," like the light, for the night. Consequently, the baby sleeping through the night has become many parents' immediate life goal. Unfortunately, this goal has become big business for the hosts of "baby sleep trainers" who promote various versions of "controlled crying" or "crying-it-out solutions."

## Breastsleeping

For new mothers, sleep and feeding are completely intertwined; it makes no sense to talk about one without the other. Feeding method influences how long babies sleep and how often they wake. When speaking about breastfeeding mothers, mother-baby sleep expert, Dr. James McKenna found that sleep and breastfeeding were so interconnected that he coined a new word: breastsleeping. Breastsleeping is sleeping by breastfeeding and breastfeeding while sleeping.

Contrary to sleeping through the night, James McKenna explains that night waking while breastsleeping is *good*. It protects babies from SIDS because:

- The baby gets to be checked,
- The baby absorbs all sorts of stimuli from the mother, such as her breathing out carbon dioxide, which helps the baby to breathe more continuously,
- The baby absorbs her smell, touch, warmth, and the movement of her chest,
- The baby spends the night in safer, *lighter sleep*,
- The baby grows specific brain architecture, and
- The baby's lighter sleep terminates apneas (abnormal cessation of breathing, of more than 20 seconds), which occur during too-deep sleep.

In fact, deep sleep and sleeping through the night are not good for babies. A prominent theory of SIDS is that babies go into such deep sleep that they cannot rouse themselves. In other words, it is for a baby's health and survival to learn to sleep *lightly and to awaken quickly, than to learn to sleep deeply without waking up. "Sensory deprivation" and "arousal deficiency" is what happens to babies who are missing the stimulation the mother's body provides.*

In a laboratory study, mothers experienced 30% more arousals when they slept with their infants (Mosko, Richard, & McKenna, 1997b). Mother-infant pairs tended to sleep in synchrony, with more than 70% of their arousals overlapping (Mosko, Richard, & McKenna, 1997a). Moreover, mothers who bedshared checked on their babies more frequently during the night. In Baddock and colleagues' study (2006), bedsharing mothers checked on their babies a median of 11 times. For mothers sleeping in separate beds, the median was 4 times (Baddock, Galland, Boltan, Williams, & Taylor, 2006).

When parents accept that night waking is normal and good, parents sleep better because they stop their endless struggle to "create good sleeping habits." What really keeps parents awake at night is worrying that there is something intrinsically wrong with their baby or toddler who keeps waking up at night. They are trying fix something that is not broken.

## Babies Need Contact with Their Mothers

The myth of "sleeping through the night" prevents us from asking the most essential question: "What sort of sleeping arrangement makes babies feel best?" Throughout pregnancy, *the babies'* well-being is regulated by their mothers' bodies—babies are in constant physical contact with their mothers, receives sensory input from them, are rocked to sleep by them, and are awake when their mothers are motionless.

Many health professionals may believe that newborns no longer need to be in constant contact with their mothers, but they are mistaken. We somehow think that babies are spoiled or have developed a bad habit when they express this most basic biological need. We expect independence from newborns or 4-month-old babies. "Sleeping through the night" and "self-soothing" were two concepts that appeared because of formula, which enabled both daytime and nighttime separation of mothers and babies. Biology, however, does not change as quickly as culture.

### Can Babies Sleep at the Breast?

Health professionals, and other parents, also make new parents feel guilty for letting their babies fall asleep at the breast. Our culture thinks that babies should fall asleep on their own and learn to "self-soothe." Breastfeeding, however, puts *both the mother and baby* to sleep. It is normal for mothers to feel drowsy towards the end of the feeding and for babies to fall asleep at the breast. Many parents get frustrated when they try to "break" this sleep association. In many languages of the world, the word breastfeeding translates as "calming down" or "quiet down"—all references to how breast-feeding enables babies' transition from wakeful to asleep.

The need to suck to fall asleep is obvious to parents, which is why so many use pacifiers as a substitute for the breast. This has reached absurd proportions when people say, "The baby is using me as a pacifier." In fact, the breastsleeping baby is only doing what his innate physiology is telling him to do—falling asleep by breastfeeding.

## Why Sleep-Deprived Parents Turn to Formula

Sleep deprivation figures prominently in reasons families give for supple-menting with formula or even stopping breastfeeding completely. Formula companies try to convince new parents that formula is the answer to all their "sleep problems." Unfortunately, parents believe the siren call of the formula companies. Pediatricians may also chime in, repeating many of the same myths. This translates into behavior. For example,

⚫ Many parents give their babies a bottle of formula to get them to sleep at night.

⚫ Sleeping through the night is why parents night wean or stop breastfeeding altogether.

⚫ Some parents "top up" with formula after a breastfeed to get the baby to fall asleep.

⚫ Some fathers or other family members bottle-feed breastfed babies at night so that the breastfeeding mother may get some sleep. This is very common in our experience.

⚫ Some parents worry that the baby is not getting enough milk in case the baby does not fall asleep once they have breastfed.

⚫ Parents think that babies sleeping for a longer stretch means they got enough to eat. If the baby wakes up after a 20- or 40-minute nap, it is taken as a sign of "low milk supply."

In reality, topping up with formula does not lead to better sleep for either mothers or babies. Three different research studies show that exclusively breastfeeding mothers get *more* sleep, have more energy, and better overall wellbeing than mothers who are mixed or formula-feeding (Doan, Gardiner, Gay, & Lee, 2007; Dorheim, Bondevik, Eberhard-Gran, & Bjorvatn, 2009; Kendall-Tackett, Cong, & Hale, 2011). Exclusively breastfeeding mothers are still tired (postpartum is hard), but they are less tired than mothers who use formula. Consistently, when mothers in these studies used formula, they were more (not less) tired.

Interestingly the exclusively breastfeeding mothers are also waking more often, and their babies sleep for shorter amounts of time at the longest stretch (Kendall-Tackett et al., 2011). What accounts for these seemingly contradictory findings? It likely has to do with the hormones of breastfeeding making it easier for exclusively breastfeeding mothers to get back to sleep and, in many cases, not even having to completely wake up to feed their babies. When babies need formula, someone must wake completely, turn on a light, and prepare a bottle. Once you do that, it's much more difficult to go quickly back to sleep.

## How Breastfeeding Mothers Can Cope with Fatigue

Although breastfeeding helps mothers get more sleep than mothers who use formula, interrupted sleep can still be a challenge. Parents may also worry that they are doing something wrong, especially if their babies are not sleeping through the night. The truth is that most babies take months, or even years, to sleep through the night. That is normal but other parents may not tell them the truth. Sometimes, just knowing the truth can keep parents from worrying that they are doing something wrong. The goal is for parents to have accurate knowledge about how babies sleep and to provide them with some ways of coping with disrupted sleep. Below are some tips to make parents' coping with sleep disruptions a bit easier.

### How to Help a Baby Sleep

Babies need help to fall asleep. Expecting babies to "self-soothe" and magically fall asleep on their own leads to lots of crying. Parents hope that their babies will somehow know that they need to fall asleep. What can parents do?

◆ Allow babies to fall asleep at the breast once they have breastfed well. Babies will usually gently release the breast as they fall into deeper asleep.

◆ Mothers can take the baby to bed with them, breastfeed lying down, and let them fall asleep.

◆ Mothers should wait until babies are really asleep (this may take much longer than most parents expect). Do *not* ease a sucking baby off the breast before they are asleep as they will wake up again. Once they stop sucking, they will eventually allow the breast out of their mouth.

◆ Walk babies to sleep in a carrier or a wrap. Breastfeeding them at the same time helps, as does walking outside.

◆ Put babies to sleep before they are too tired and overstimulated.

◆ Use vertical motion (up and down) to help babies quiet down and fall asleep. One way to do this is for parents to use a big exercise ball to gently rock the baby up and down.

◆ Parents should make sure babies get enough total sleep time. Some parents try to have their babies sleep as little as possible during the day hoping they will sleep better at night. However, babies need good sleep both during the day and at night. Keeping babies up longer during the day does not work.

◆ Just as breastfeeding and sleeping are interconnected, so are sleep and brain development. Lighter sleep and frequent night-time waking are connected to memory formation and brain development.

◆ Skin-to-skin contact helps babies calm down and fall asleep because it increases the amount of oxytocin in both mother and baby.

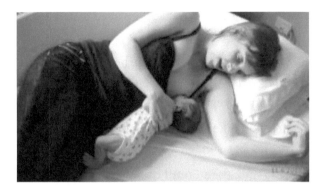

This mother is feeding her baby lying down, side by side with her baby. Well-latched babies often seem to get more milk when they are feeding side by side with the mother as in the photo. This works particularly well when the mother has less milk, as in the evening. Generally, babies seem calmer in this position, particularly in the evening.

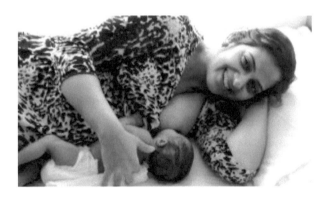

Lying side by side and feeding the baby is a good way for the mother to rest and to sleep together with the baby.

## This, Too, Shall Pass

Eventually, all babies sleep through the night and fall asleep on their own. This happens without letting them cry it out. They simply "grow up" and their sleep patterns naturally change. There is no reason for night weaning to achieve sleeping through the night. Nighttime breastfeeding provides babies with security and helps them transition from one sleep cycle to the next. Statistically speaking, the overall length of breastfeeding depends on the baby and toddler breastfeeding at night. In the meantime, there are things mothers can do now to help them cope with frequent night wakings.

- Accept that this is normal. Parents are not doing anything wrong.

- Make sure that both mother and baby have a comfortable sleeping space. If the bed is too small or mothers worry that their babies might fall out of bed, mothers will sleep less well than they should. Putting a mattress on the floor and sleeping there with the baby may help a lot.

- Know that night wakings help their babies' brain to develop.

- Stop counting the times the baby woke up at night. If the parents avoid the counting, nighttime harmony will develop in which the mother will wake up a few seconds before the baby, put the baby to the breast, and continue sleeping almost without noticing the interruption.

- Stop giving bottles to let mothers get more sleep. This does not work. When families in our clinic try it, no one gets much sleep. Bottles interrupt nighttime harmony. In the long run, giving bottles to the baby at night also lowers mothers' milk production because some babies get a lot of their breastmilk intake at night. Sleeping with the baby at night increases the number of times the baby breastfeeds, which increases mothers' milk supply.

- Start breastfeeding the baby as soon as the baby stirs instead of waiting for full-blown crying, which may make babies too upset to eat. They must be calmed down first.

- Know that the average sleep cycle of a baby at night is about 90 minutes.

- Try to sleep as soon as the baby sleeps at night instead of using the first sleep to stay up.

## When Doctors Recommend Sleep Training

When exhausted parents turn to their doctors, doctors try to "fix" normal sleep patterns by recommending sleep training. This anti-nature idea is extremely attractive to many parents; they can "do" something to make themselves less tired. What is more appealing than several uninterrupted hours of sleep? Other parents may be convinced sleep training is part of being a good parent, even when it feels wrong to them.

Professional sleep trainers are doing a booming trade by forcing babies to sleep through the night at physiologically inappropriate ages. Sleep trainers spend nights letting babies cry so that the "learn" not to wake up and breastfeed. This sometimes "works," and babies appear to sleep longer. Some trainers even get very young babies to sleep through the night, but at what cost? Even the Hospital for Sick Children (Toronto), not exactly a gushing fountain of knowledge and understanding about breastfeeding, will not see babies younger than 6-months-of-age for night waking "issues."

### The Problem with Sleep Training

The problem with sleep training—and it is a big problem—is its negative effect on breastfeeding. Night feedings maintain mothers' milk supply. Furthermore, if their milk supply and flow decreases for whatever reason, the *best* feedings, sometimes the *only* feedings, occur at night. Sleep trainers may also introduce pacifiers, which can also negatively affect breastfeeding. Unfortunately, sleep training frequently means the end of breastfeeding.

Milk supply is not the only problem. Babies learn to trust others by trusting their mothers. What do babies learn when no one comes when they cry? Answer: that no one cares how desperate they get. Trust is lost.

In our view, leaving babies to cry isn't good from any angle. Sleep training is highly stressful for babies. It increases babies' levels of the stress hormone cortisol. High cortisol levels not only suppress the immune system, making babies more vulnerable to illness, but it is specifically toxic to brain cells and can impact learning and memory (Sapolsky, 1996).

One well-publicized sleep-training study found that sleep training was "not harmful." However, they also found "no benefits." It did not reduce mothers' risk of depression or improve infant sleep (Price, Wake, Ukoumunne, & Hiscock, 2012). Why do it, then? Why expose babies to toxic levels of stress hormones? Surely, no good comes from that. In conclusion, we do not accept that "crying it out" can be a part of good parenting.

## Conclusion

Breastfeeding and sleep are so interwoven that Dr. James McKenna calls it "breastsleeping." Feeding babies frequently at night protects them from SIDS. Current sleep-training recommendations do not improve infant sleep or mother's fatigue. However, these measures negatively affect her milk supply and involve breaking trust with their infants. We do not recommend sleep training and believe that it is harmful.

# CHAPTER 23

# How Long Is It Normal to Breastfeed?

Let us say a mother has defied the odds and has breastfed her baby exclusively for 6 months. She has hit a significant milestone. Unfortunately, rather than congratulating her, people start pressuring her to stop. It could be subtle. They may ask, "how long do you intend to keep *that* up"? Many times, the pressure is not at all subtle. It can come from friends and relatives, health professionals, strangers, and even the mother's partner. Everyone, it seems, has an opinion on how long it is appropriate to breastfeed.

The attitude frequently is, "You've done your duty; you've breastfed exclusively for 6 months. Isn't that enough?" The people asking are often surprised when mothers tell them that they never considered breastfeeding a "duty." That they liked, even loved, breastfeeding and so did their babies. Why should they stop? Breastfeeding may have started as a duty, but it's not that way now. Mothers in our clinic tell us that they love breastfeeding, especially if they have overcome difficulties.

The WHO recommends breastfeeding for *at least* 2 years, but that age continues to shock North Americans. The American Academy of Pediatrics recommends breastfeeding for at least 12 months and *as long as the mother and baby mutually desire.* Some physicians, even ones who support breastfeeding, argue that breastfeeding is the normal way of feeding *babies,* but there should be a limit.

## Is Breastfeeding Past One Year Harmful?

We regularly receive questions about this. Many healthcare providers tell mothers that there is "no point in breastfeeding past 1 year." Beyond that, many believe that breastfeeding past a certain age is weird and even wrong, that it's more about the *mother's* needs than those of her infant or toddler.

## "Sexual, Sinful, and Shameful"

The American Academy of Pediatrics modified the WHO's recommendation of breastfeeding to 2 years and beyond. Perhaps members of the Academy knew that American pediatricians would not support breastfeeding to age 2 *and beyond*, so they recommended 12 months and for as long as the mother and child desire. Even with that change, the backlash was swift and severe. Popular media and journalists in the United States were horrified by the notion of breastfeeding to 12 months. Longer was unthinkable. We've now had 25 years to adjust to the recommended 12 months. That "might" be okay, but longer than that? Why?

The reader might be wondering that yourself. If that is the case, please suspend skepticism for a bit as we explore the possibility of breastfeeding past 12 months and even to 2 years and beyond. It is not harmful and if the mother and baby have gone to a year, and it is often a delight for mother and baby. Is it a sin? Some people, including many doctors would say "yes."

As we have said repeatedly, breastfeeding is not just about *breastmilk*; it's a *relationship*. We sometimes use the analogy of a couple unable to have children. Nobody tells them, we assume, not to make love, because if you cannot make a baby, what is the point? The point is the same with breastfeeding. It's about a physical and emotional relationship between two people who love each other.

What happens if children do not want to stop at 12 months? Forcing a 12-month-old to stop breastfeeding based on an arbitrary "recommended" age is usually much harder work than allowing that child to continue doing what makes that child happy. Trying to prevent toddlers from breastfeeding often makes them extremely upset. When this happens, mothers are advised to "just let them cry it out. They will eventually 'get it.'" Yes, probably they will eventually "get it," but at what price? This approach is extremely difficult not only for the child, but also the parents and other children as well. Maybe it would be fine if the child cried for

5 minutes (though we do not agree). Many will cry for a much longer time. They can break your heart. I (JN) remember we did this with our oldest son. He would wake up several times in the night and one time, we decided, "no, we will let him wait." After about 20 horrible minutes (not only for him) of this 3-year-old crying, he said, standing in his crib, "This is your little boy Daniel, why are you doing this?" It was the last time we used the crib. Daniel continued to breastfeed until he was almost 4 and then he stopped on his own.

### Is Breastfeeding a 3- Or 4-Year-Old Sexual?

This question is important to address directly. Many 3 or even 4-year-old children still drink from a bottle, especially at night to help them fall asleep and fall asleep again if they wake. What does it mean, if someone considers a 3- or 4-year-old sucking milk from a bottle acceptable or even normal, but considers another 3- or 4-year-old breastfeeding to be "overdependent"? More disturbing, does breastfeeding indicate a "sexual relationship between the mother and child"?

As outrageous as this idea is, it is something that some professionals believe. One pediatric psychiatrist in France considers breastfeeding a child older than 7 months to be sexual abuse. In an interview, he said, "When a child touches his mother's breasts, she should say to him 'No, leave me alone. These are your daddy's and mommy's toys. You have your toy car" (*L'Express*, October 9, 2003). We are without words. Perhaps this psychiatrist is being deliberately provocative, but it seems unlikely as he is known for repeating such inane remarks frequently and thus this was not a one-off remark in a hotly discussed interview.

Why do so many in industrialized cultures think that breastfeeding a 3-year-old is sexual? It might have to do with the idea that the breasts themselves are seen as primarily sexual. Check any number of men's magazines. Yes, infants can derive nourishment from the breast, but there comes a time that a child no longer "needs" the breast for nourishment. The child psychiatrist mentioned above thinks that time limit is 7 months of age.

Another test of "too old" is when they can ask for it. It's a strange thing to say because even newborns are very good at "asking" for breastfeeding. They just don't use words. Very young infants root, looking for the breast. If they're not given the breast soon enough, they will begin to cry. The young toddler may have "baby" words for the breast but is still "asking for it." And some babies have learned sign language. You know what? An 8-month-old can ask for the breast with sign language! So, the 8-month-old is asking for the breast, though non-verbally. How does being verbal change this whole relationship of breastfeeding into something abnormally "sexual"?

## Does Breastfeeding Past 12 Months Harm Children's Development?

Some people think that breastfeeding past 12 months is harmful and "gross," and are often forceful in their opinions. Even strangers in public places will weigh in. Mothers often respond to this by going underground and secretly continue breastfeeding. They often develop codewords for breastfeeding so if they are not alone, the child can ask for it without revealing the truth.

One of the largest public assaults on "prolonged breastfeeding" happened in 2012, when *Time Magazine* published an article called: Are You Mom Enough? The cover showing a mother breastfeeding a 3-year-old, who, because of his standing position looked much older. There is something so terribly wrong about the title itself. It is a title that is likely to infuriate many mothers, implying that if they did not breastfeed for 3 years, they are not good enough mothers. It seems to us that this title was deliberately chosen to be provocative. The letters to the editor undoubtedly came in by the thousands. Some were likely supportive, many undoubtedly not. A male journalist in Toronto, writing in the "subway free newspaper" could only comment "prepare the psychiatrist's couch." I was uncertain if he meant for the child or the mother.

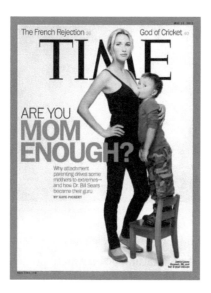

Breastfeeding a toddler, or an even older child, has become common enough in most resource- rich countries that people no longer consider it *that* odd. Issues do arise, nevertheless, as the *Time* story suggests. Few people will support a mother if she wishes to breastfeed for 4 years or more. Friends and family will tell them that they are damaging their child by breastfeeding for such a long time, that the child will be a mocked, insecure, "momma's boy" (*especially* if the child is a boy).

Older children undoubtedly love breastfeeding. Anyone who observes older children without prejudice will see that they are very relaxed and content to be at the breast. Mothers will tell you that it is a great way to calm an upset child, regardless of the reason for their being upset, and that they consider it an essential part of their relationship with their child.

The reassuring fact is that all children eventually stop breastfeeding—guaranteed. A day will come when the mother realizes that her child did not breastfeed during the night, the last breastfeed that most young children give up on their own.

Do nursing 5-year-olds still receive milk or are they "using the mother as a pacifier"? Clearly, if one looks, the child is receiving milk. Is that milk still good? Of course.

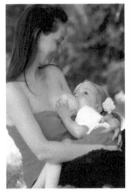
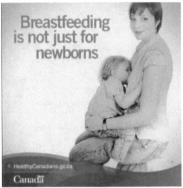

These photos show children, who are clearly not infants, breastfeeding. The photo on the right is of a Canadian government poster. If this disturbs your doctor, tell him/her to get over it.

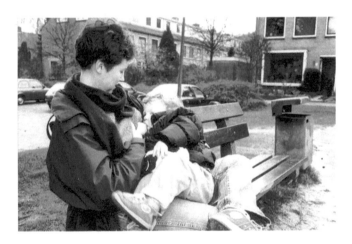

In the photo above, the child is clearly not a newborn. This mother is breast-feeding on a day that is clearly not sunny and warm. Still, the milk will be warm enough.

### Burdensome to Families

Another concern is that breastfeeding past 12 months burdens mothers and the rest of the family. That breastfeeding toddlers are demanding. That they expect to be breastfed frequently even though they are also eating food. It might help to remember that *all* babies, toddlers, and children older than toddlers can be demanding. They all want their parents' attention frequently, not only when they are unhappy. This is true even if they are no longer breastfeeding.

When babies or toddlers are unhappy, the breast provides a quick fix—a *good* quick fix. But many health professionals unfortunately call it, "an unhealthy fix." Obviously, we disagree. Is picking up the unhappy child, hugging, and consoling them unhealthy? Most health professionals would say that it is not, but add breastfeeding to the mix, and suddenly it is. Let us face it; many pediatricians are uncomfortable with breastfeeding. Mothers tell us that very few pediatricians ever observed them feeding at the breast. So, we should not be surprised when they are uncomfortable with breastfeeding an unhappy toddler.

There are, obviously, situations when it would be inappropriate for the child to have the breast immediately. For example, when mothers are driving with their child sitting in the car seat. However, even on a motorway, there are usually places to stop safely, so the child may just have to wait for a while. Mothers can also gently teach older babies and toddlers not to lift their shirts in public.

### Frequent Night Waking

Continued night waking is another reason why people are concerned about toddler breastfeeding. This issue can be difficult for parents. Night waking will not be true for *all* breastfeeding toddlers, but it can definitely be an issue for some. Night waking is *also* true for non-breastfeeding babies and toddlers, which explains why many are kept asleep with pacifiers or propped bottles of formula or sweetened water. See the chapter on sleep.

In colonial North American, parents and their children still slept together, often all in one bed. As industrialization influenced almost every aspect of life, parents and children were advised to sleep separately. Even so, many mothers still slept with their babies. In the late 20th century pediatricians warned parents not to sleep with their babies, especially when they are younger than 6 months of age, because they believed it increased the risk of SIDS (sudden infant death syndrome). For exclusively breastfed babies, bedsharing lowers the risk of SIDS if there are no other environmental risks, such as parents who smoke or use mind-altering substances, and there is no fluffy bedding or places for babies to get wedged (McKenna, 2020). Even if babies are not breastfed, they should still sleep in the parents' room, but not in the same bed, for the first 6 months of life to lower their risk of SIDS.

If mothers co-sleep with their babies, they often will not wake up at all when babies search for the breast and latch on. More likely, mothers briefly wake up but then fall back to sleep, and so will the child. Night feedings are particularly important to toddlers. They are usually the last feedings that they give up when they are in the sometimes-long process of stopping breastfeeding. We are all more or less afraid of the dark, but young children are especially so. Breastfeeding reassures them that all is well.

## Tooth Decay

Some dentists believe that breastfed toddlers are more likely to get tooth decay. They think that breastfeeding a toddler at night is like leaving a toddler with a bottle of formula or sugar water. The two situations are not equivalent. Babies left with bottles of formula or sugar water have the liquid in their mouths bathing the teeth for long periods of time in the night. Breastfeeding babies may breastfeed many times during the night, though only minutes at a time.

Unlike the situation when the bottle leaks milk continuously into babies' mouths, with sugary fluid (and that includes formula) in continuous contact with babies' teeth, when the toddler is breastfeeding, the nipple is well back in babies' mouths, away from the front teeth, which are most likely to be damaged. Furthermore, the milk is swallowed and does not bathe the toddler's teeth. It is believed that those breastfed babies who do develop cavities, do so because the teeth were damaged in utero, probably due to some febrile illness of the mother during the pregnancy. In any case, with time, baby teeth are replaced with adult teeth and in our experience, the adult teeth are not damaged by what happened to the baby teeth.

## Conclusion

The World Health Organization (World Health Organization, 2021), and most pediatric organizations around the world, recommend breastfeeding to 2 years and *beyond* with no upper limit mentioned. This is not just for the developing world or resource-poor societies. WHO speaks for the whole world. And many people in resource-rich countries who do not share the wealth of those societies.

Breastfeeding is good for children's health at any age. Two-year-olds are often in contact with many other children. Daycare centers are often sites of mini epidemics of diarrhea, colds, and parasites in the bowels (*Giardia lamblia*). Breastfeeding protects children from infections at any age, and even should they be infected, their illnesses are usually much less severe.

For most families who breastfeed past 12 months, health is one factor. The other is their relationship with their child. Breastfeeding is a way to comfort a frightened or hurt or frustrated child that works like a charm. Many mothers consider it their secret weapon.

CHAPTER 24

# Breastfeeding Myths That Even Some Lactation Consultants Believe

This book has focused on health professionals and what they know about breastfeeding. Lactation consultants are generally the most knowledgeable supporters of breastfeeding and frequently advise other health professionals. We are confident that they are aware of many of the topics we have discussed. We also hope that they learned something new in reading through this book. However, there are a few more issues for us to discuss. Over the years, we've been surprised that even some lactation consultants have learned inaccurate things about breastfeeding. You might disagree with what we say in this chapter, but we ask you to consider suspending your skepticism to see if what we say makes sense. Myths are transferred from generation to generation, so if something is not correct based on what we know now, it's a good to change course.

## 1. Babies Transfer Milk (No, They Do Not)

If babies transfer milk, it follows that they must "work hard" to suck the milk out of the breast. This construct has a lot of implications for practice. We have observed that most health professionals have forgotten why they think breastfeeding is hard work for the baby, but they just accept the notion. This notion resonates throughout pediatric hospital wards, but particularly in the neonatal intensive care unit (NICU), where it leads to policies such as not letting babies breastfeed until 34 weeks gestation.

Consider a baby waking from sleep. The baby begins to move and show signs of hunger. The mother's mind, body, and breasts react. The mother has a milk-ejection reflex, and the front of her blouse becomes wet. Who transferred the milk? Obviously, the mother did. She transferred the milk on to her clothes, and not into the baby's mouth. (Using the expression "transfer milk" has always seemed odd to us. We transfer funds or a baton in a foot race. We transfer from the bus to the subway. But milk?)

Who stimulated the mother's milk-ejection reflex? Babies, of course, just as they do when they are latched on and suckle. They are not passive vessels who just receive the milk, but they do not suck milk out of the breast and are not working hard.

## Babies are Often Blamed

I (JN) have heard other conference speakers who blame babies for falling asleep at the breast. For example, one speaker said that near-term babies do not breastfeed well because their "cheek muscles" are not well developed. This is the height of absurdity. Premature babies can latch on and breast-feed at 28 weeks, but 36-week gestation babies cannot? Because they have undeveloped cheek muscles?

Sometimes, mothers are told that their babies are lazy, or that the baby has a "high palate," "bubble palate," or that the baby is "an impatient baby," or a "baby does not know what to do." When professionals believe that babies transfer milk, babies get blamed for all sorts of things without being offered any solutions.

## Milk Flow vs. Hard Work

In our view, babies are more likely to fall asleep at the breast when milk flow slows, especially if they are younger than 2 months of age. As they get older, they tend to pull off the breast when the flow slows down. If sleeping babies are then taken off the breast before they have had a full feed, they will search for the breast or start to cry. The slow flow at the breast has the same effect on the baby as the pacifier. Unlike with a pacifier, the mother *may* have another milk-ejection reflex, but usually the milk ejection will be smaller and shorter. If the mother changes sides when the baby is starting to fall asleep, the baby will often wake up on the second breast and drink very well, even with open eyes. This emphasizes the point that babies respond to milk flow and that breastfeeding is not the "hard work" of sucking milk out of the breast.

This video demonstrates the fallacy of believing that babies transfer milk. The baby in the video was born at 35 weeks gestation. Typically, as in far too many NICUs, the mother did not get good advice and help with breastfeeding and she did not get help to latch the baby on, the most critical skill. The first problem was the baby being sent to the NICU, since the baby was born at 35 weeks gestation but did not have any medical problems. Why was the baby in the NICU? The mother did not know.

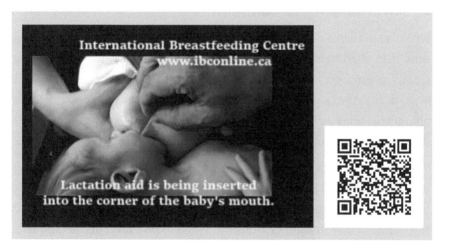

We see the baby at 5 weeks of age, so 40 weeks "gestation" now. The baby has fallen asleep at the breast *because the flow of milk had slowed, not because sucking was hard work*. The mother tries breast compressions, but the compressions are not helping get the baby more milk at this point. The baby falls back to sleep and does not even suck.

The tube of the lactation aid is introduced, which stimulates the baby to suck, but as there is still no flow (the milk just reaches the baby's mouth but stops there), the baby falls asleep again. The tube is adjusted, so that the baby gets milk with sucking. He starts to drink and opens his eyes wide. We think this is good proof that, at least in this case, that it was not "hard work" that made the baby fall asleep from fatigue, but rather the lack of milk flow.

### Use Breast Compressions to Increase Flow

To increase milk flow, we generally recommend starting breast compressions when the flow of milk has started to slow but not almost stopped. Breast compressions, if done properly (though not a complicated technique) will keep the baby drinking by augmenting the flow of milk and the baby will stay awake, drinking longer.

## 2. "Oversupply" is Common

In our experience, "oversupply" rarely exists. Lactation consultants diagnose this when babies cough and choke at the breast as they are feeding. Coughing and choking, however, does not prove that there is *too much milk,* or that the flow is so rapid that the baby cannot keep up. Oversupply also gets diagnosed if the mother's breasts are constantly "full" or she gets recurrent blocked ducts or mastitis.

If babies cannot handle the flow, or mothers report that they are constantly full, the real problem is that the baby's latch is not as good as it could be. We know it sounds like we are saying that a less-than-adequate latch is the source of *almost* all breastfeeding problems. We say it because it's true.

Why is the baby's latch not good? Technique, Technique, Technique. (Also, use of bottles, pacifiers). Another possibility is that the baby has a tongue-tie. We diagnose tongue-ties on the basis of poor "vertical lift" of the tongue + mother's symptoms (*the* most important), not how well babies can stick out their tongues.

Diagnosing "oversupply" leads to recommendations with which we just do not agree, such as, offering only one breast at each feed, even several feeds on same side ("block feeding"), the use of nipple shields to "slow the flow," or doing "feeding" studies of the baby "choking at the breast." All of these recommendations decrease milk supply. The baby might also be wrongly diagnosed with "reflux," colic, or allergy to cows'-milk protein (or soy protein, etc., etc.), which results in restricting the mother's diet and frequently, "special formulas" for baby.

Fix how the baby latches on, and there is likely to be no more "oversupply."

## 3. Pumping Accurately Measures Supply

Pumping, much beloved by many lactation consultants, does not tell us anything about how much the baby gets from the breast. A baby who is well latched on is likely to receive more milk than a mother can pump. A baby who is poorly latched on will likely receive less than the mother can pump.

Some mothers are advised to pump between feedings. This seems to get them more milk, but at the next feeding, the baby may get less milk, if it is only, say 2 hours after the pumping.

A better approach is for the mother to receive good help and, possibly, start domperidone depending on the situation and observation of the feeding. The baby will get more milk from the breast, but because of that, the mother may get less when she pumps.

It is not rare for us to receive questions from mothers wondering why the domperidone decreased their milk production. By only looking at pumping, practitioners get a false picture of what is happening. Domperidone does not always increase what the baby receives from the breast, but it does not decrease it, unless, for some reason the baby's latch gets worse (more bottles?).

In other words, what the mother pumps does not tell the mother or the lactation consultant what the baby gets from the breast.

## 4. Test Weighing Is a Good Way to Know If the Baby Is Getting Enough

Weighing a baby before and after a breastfeeding, called test weighing or weighted feeds, is a method that is used to determine whether the baby is getting enough milk from the breast. At first glance, looking at test weights seems scientific and accurate, but it is not. In the first place, the amount that the baby "needs" at a feeding is based on formula-feeding norms. Even formula-fed babies do not always drink the same amount at every feed.

Breastmilk is not the same as formula and there is no evidence for this assumption that the "standard" amount of formula a baby requires determines how much breastmilk the baby requires. Furthermore, breastmilk quantities ingested by the baby, can vary from feeding to feeding, not only in volume, but also in its various components, especially fat (Paulaviciene, Liubsys, Molyte, Eidukaite, & Usonis, 2020). Perhaps 20 ml (2/3 ounce) of higher-fat milk may be as adequate as 30 ml of lower-fat milk or 30 ml of formula. Fat content also varies during a single feeding, and from day to day (Mitoulas et al., 2002). Test weighing will not reflect the differences in fat content. If the milk is higher fat, a smaller volume may be enough.

The volume of breastmilk ingested by the baby may have nothing to do with the baby's satisfaction. Maybe something else determines why babies seem to "need" more milk in the evening. Hahn-Holbrook and colleagues (2019) suggest that what a mother expresses depends on the time of day. Not only do the amounts vary, but so do the components of breastmilk. Also, most mothers will agree that they seem to have more milk in the morning than in the evening, and the baby *seems* to be more satisfied from a morning breastfeed. Thus, if the milk intake is measured in the morning, the result may be falsely reassuring. If measured in the late afternoon or evening, the result may be falsely concerning.

Anxiety can suppress the milk-ejection reflex and thus, how much milk the baby will receive from the breast. Test weighings can cause anxiety and may limit how much milk mothers can pump or, in the case of test weighing, how much the baby receives from the breast. Stress inhibits many bodily functions. For example, "Please pee in this jar while the police officer watches you."

## 5. Breastmilk in a Bottle Is the Same as Breastfeeding

We are sorry to have to write this, as mothers already feel bad enough if they try to save their breastfeeding by bottle-feeding breastmilk. They hate to hear that breastfeeding differs from feeding breastmilk in the bottle. They usually know that this is true, even if only subliminally. So many mothers that we see want to get their babies off the bottle, or off the nipple shield, even though, at least for the moment, breastmilk feeding results in the baby gaining well and the mothers "accept," sort of, these methods of feeding.

Breastfeeding is a close, intimate, physical, and emotional relationship between two (sometimes three) people who love each other. This does not mean that mothers cannot have close intimate relationships with their bottle-feeding babies. They certainly can, but we should not pretend that feeding method does not influence the relationship. Mothers understand this intrinsically. In general, mothers want to stop using bottles when they are supplementing. They want to get rid of the nipple shield. Unfortunately, they are not always aware that something can be done. Neither are most health professionals aware that something can be done.

Even if it is necessary to supplement, supplementation can and should be given by lactation aid at the breast. If the mother supplements at the breast, she is still breastfeeding, even breastfeeding *exclusively*. True, the baby may not receive only breastmilk if the mother uses the lactation aid at the breast and supplements with formula, but she and the baby are still breastfeeding.

*Breastfeeding exclusively?* We think they are because we are focusing on the act of breastfeeding and the relationship, not just the milk. If the mother must give formula, she needs good hands-on help to breastfeed as much as possible, at the breast.

Mothers can also get donated breastmilk. There are websites where this can be arranged. Mothers should not pay for the breastmilk! When money comes into the picture, there is a possibility of corruption such as adding formula to the breastmilk, to make a "little extra." Furthermore, the mother donating the milk and the mother receiving the milk for her baby should live close enough so that the milk can be delivered in person. We feel that such an "intimate" gift requires person-to-person contact.

## Conclusion

We have many years of clinical experience and have lived long enough to see various fads in the lactation world. We are both concerned about some of the information taught at lactation conferences or things that mothers have told us. Many of these theories, or methods of doing things, make breastfeeding more difficult, or leads to policies that can have a severe negative impact. We want to pass along what we have learned and hope that it will help you in your personal breastfeeding journey or your clinical practice.

# References

Ahluwalia, I. B., Morrow, B., & Hsia, J. (2005). Why do women stop breastfeeding? Findings from the Pregnancy Risk Assessment and Monitoring System. *Pediatrics, 116*(6), 1408-1412. doi:10.1542/peds.2005-0013

American College of Radiologists. (2021). ACR manual on contrast media. Retrieved from https://www.acr.org/-/media/ACR/files/clinical-resources/contrast_media.pdf

Armstrong, J., Reilly, J. J., & The Child Health Information Team. (2002). Breastfeeding and lowering the risk of childhood obesity. *Lancet, 359*, 2003-2004.

Aronsson, C. A., Lee, H.-S., Liu, E., Uusitalo, U., Hummel, S., Yang, J., . . . The TEDDY Study Group. (2015). Age at gluten introduction and risk of celiac disease. *Pediatrics, 135*(2), 239-245. doi:10.1542/peds.2014-1787

Babic, A., Sasamoto, N., Rosner, B. A., Tworoger, S. S., Jordan, S. J., & Risch, H. A. (2020). Association between breastfeeding and ovarian cancer risk. *JAMA Oncology, 6*(6), e200421. doi:10.1001/jamaoncol.2020.0421

Baddock, S. A., Galland, B. C., Boltan, D. P., Williams, S. M., & Taylor, B. J. (2006). Differences in infant and parent behaviors during routine bed sharing compared with cot sleeping in the home setting. *Pediatrics, 117*(5), 1599-1607. doi:10.1542/peds.2005-1636

Bartick, M., & Reinhold, A. (2010). The burden of suboptimal breastfeeding in the United States: A pediatric cost analysis. *Pediatrics, 125*, e1048. doi:10.1542/peds.2009-161

Beilin, Y., Bodian, C. A., Weiser, J., Hossain, S., Arnold, I., Feierman, D. E., . . . Holzman, I. (2005). Effect on labor epidural analgesia with and without fentanyl on infant breastfeeding: A prospective, randomized, double-blind study. *Anesthesiology, 103*(6), 1211-1217.

Bergman, N. J., Linley, L. L., & Fawcus, S. R. (2004). Randomized controlled trial of skin-to-skin contact from birth versus conventional incubator form physiological stabilization in 1200- to 2199-gram newborns. *Acta Paediatrica, 93*, 779-785. doi:10.1080/08035250410028534

Bever, L. (2017). She listened to her doctors--and her baby died. Now she's warning others about breastfeeding. *Washington Post.* Retrieved from https://www.washingtonpost.com/news/parenting/wp/2017/03/08/she-listened-to-her-doctors-and-her-baby-died-now-shes-warning-others-about-breast-feeding/

Bigelow, J. L., Dunson, D. B., Stanford, J. B., Ecochard, R., Gnoth, C., & Colombo, B. (2004). Mucus observations in the fertile window: A better predictor of conception than timing of intercourse. *Human Reproduction, 19*(4), 889-892. doi:10.1093/humrep/deh173

Bognar, Z., DeLuca, D., Domellof, M., Hadjipanayis, A., Haffner, D., & Johnson, M. (2020). Promoting breastfeeding interaction of pediatric associations with providers of nutritional products. *Frontiers in Pediatrics, 8.* doi:https://doi.org/10.3389/fped.2020.562870

Boone, K. M., Geraghty, S. R., & Keim, S. A. (2016). Feeding at the breast and expressed milk feeding: Associations with otitis media and diarrhea in infants. *Journal of Pediatrics, 174*, 118-125. doi:https://doi.org/10.1016/j.jpeds.2016.04.006

Boostani, R., Sadeghi, R., Sabouri, A., & Ghabeli-Juibary, A. (2018). Human T-lymphotropic virus type I and breastfeeding: Systematic review and meta-analysis of the literature. *Iranian Journal of Neurology, 17*(4), 174-179. Retrieved from http://ijnl.tums.ac.ir

Borra, C., Iacovou, M., & Sevilla, A. (2015). New evidence on breastfeeding and postpartum depression: The importance of understanding women's intentions. *Maternal & Child Health Journal, 19*(4), 897-907.

Brimdyr, K., Cadwell, K., Widstrom, A.-M., Svensson, K., Neumann, M., Hart, E. A., . . . Phillips, R. (2015). The association between common labor drugs and suckling when skin to skin during the first hour after birth. *Birth, 42*(4), 319-328.

Brisbane, J. M., & Giglia, R. C. (2015). Experiences of expressing and storing colostrum antenatally: A qualitative study of mothers in regional Western Australia. *Journal of Child Health Care, 19*(2), 206-215. doi:0.1177/1367493513503586

Brown, A. E. (2019). *Why breastfeeding grief and trauma matter*. London, UK: Pinter and Martin.

Brown, C. E., & Magnuson, B. (2000). On the physics of the infant feeding bottle and middle ear sequela: Ear disease in infants can be associated with bottle feeding. *International Journal of Pediatric Otorhinolaryngology, 54*, 13-20.

Cacho, N. T., & Lawrence, R. M. (2017). Innate immunity and breast milk. *Frontiers in Immunology, 8*. doi:10.3389/fimmu.2017.00584

Canadian Agency for Drugs and Technology in Health, Palylyk-Colwell, E., & Campbell, K. (2018). Oral glucose gel for neonatal hypoglycemia: A review of clinical effectiveness, cost-effectiveness, and guidelines. Retrieved from https://www.ncbi.nlm.nih.gov/books/NBK537952/

Carneiro-Proietti, A. B. F., Seabra-Proietti, A. B. F., Amaranto-Damasio, M. S., Leal-Horiguchi, C. F., Bastos, R. H. C., Seabra-Freitas, G., & Borowiak, D. R. (2014). Mother-to-child transmission of human T-Cell lymphotropic viruses-1/2: What we know and what are the gaps in understanding and preventing this route of infection. *Journal of the Pediatric Infectious Diseases Society, 3*(Suppl 1), S24-S29. doi:10.1093/jpids/piu070

Centers for Disease Control and Prevention. (2020). Guidance: Prevention and control in peri- and postpartum settings. Retrieved from https://www.cdc.gov/flu/professionals/infectioncontrol/peri-post-settings.htm

Centers for Disease Control and Prevention. (2021). *Influenza*. Retrieved from https://www.cdc.gov/breastfeeding/breastfeeding-special-circumstances/maternal-or-infant-illnesses/influenza.html

Chantry, C. J., Nommsen-Rivers, L. A., Peerson, J. M., Cohen, R. J., & Dewey, K. G. (2011). Excess weight loss in the first-born breastfed newborns related to maternal intrapartum fluid balance. *Pediatrics, 127*, e171-e179. doi:10.1542/peds.2009-26

Charpak, N., Tessier, R., Ruiz, J. G., Hernandez, J. T., Uriza, F., Villegas, J., & Nadeau, L. (2017). Twenty-year follow-up of Kangaroo Mother Care versus traditional care. *Pediatrics, 139*(1), e20162063.

Chen, X., Chen, J., Wen, J., Chenyu, X., Zhang, S., Zhou, Y.-H., & Hu, Y. (2013). Breastfeeding is not a risk factor for mother-to-child transmission of Hepatitis B virus. *PLoS One, 8*(1), e55303. doi:10.1371/journal.pone.0055303

Chertok, I. R. A., Raz, I., Shoham, I., Haddad, H., & Wiznitzer, A. (2009). Effects of early breastfeeding on neonatal glucose levels of term infants born to women with gestational diabetes. *Journal of Human Nutrition and Dietetics, 22,* 169-169. doi:10.1111/j.1365-277X.2008.00921.x

Clarke, G., O'Mahony, S. M., Dinan, T. G., & Cryan, J. F. (2014). Priming for health: Gut microbiota acquired in early life regulates physiology, brain, and behaviour. *Acta Paediatrica, 103,* 812-819. doi:10.1111/apa.12674

Codagnone, M. G., Stanton, C., O'Mahony, S. M., Dinan, T. G., & Cryan, J. F. (2019). Microbiota and neurodevelopmental trajectories: Role of maternal and early-life nutrition. *Annals of Nutrition and Metabolism, 74*(Suppl), 16-27. doi: 10.1159/000499144

Collaborative Group on Hormonal Factors in Breast Cancer. (2002). Breast cancer and breastfeeding: Collaborative reanalysis of individual data from 47 epidemiological studies in 30 countries, including 50, 302 women with breast cancer and 96,973 women without the disease. *The Lancet, 360,* 187-195.

Conde-Agudelo, A., & Diaz-Rossello, J. L. (2014). Kangaroo mother care to reduce morbidity and mortality in low birthweight infants. *Cochrane Database of Systematic Reviews,* (4). doi:10.1002/14651858.CD002771.pub3

Cook, M. J. (2015). Lyme borreliosis: A review of data on transmission time after tick attachment. *International Journal of General Medicine, 8,* 1-5. doi:10.2147/IJGM. S73791

Cornblath, M., Hawdon, J. M., Williams, A. F., Aynsley-Green, A., Ward-Platt, M. P., Schwartz, R., & Kalhan, S. C. (2000). Controversies regarding definition of neonatal hypoglycemia: Suggested operational thresholds. *Pediatrics, 105,* 1141. doi:10.1542/ peds.105.5.1141

Dawod, B., & Marshall, J. S. (2019). Cytokines and soluble receptors in breast milk as enhancers of oral tolerance development. *Frontiers in Immunology.* Retrieved from https://doi.org/10.3389/fimmu.2019.00016

Dettwyler, K., & Stuart-McAdam, P. (1995). *Breastfeeding: Biocultural perspectives*: Aldine de Guyter.

Dhonukshe-Rutten, R. A. M., Vossenaar, M., West, C. E., Schumann, K., Bulux, J., & Solomons, N. W. (2005). Day-to-day variations in iron, zinc, and copper in breast milk of Guatemalan mothers. *Journal of Pediatric Gastroenterology and Nutrition, 40,* 128-134.

Diener, H.-C., Forderreuther, S., Gaul, C., Giese, F., Hamann, T., Holle-Lee, D., & Jurgens, T. P. (2020). Prevention of migraine with monoclonal antibodies against CGRP and the CGRP receptor. *Neurological Research and Practice, 2,* 11. doi:https://neurolrespract. biomedcentral.com/articles/10.1186/s42466-020-00057-1

Doan, T., Gardiner, A., Gay, C. L., & Lee, K. A. (2007). Breastfeeding increases sleep duration of new parents. *Journal of Perinatal & Neonatal Nursing, 21*(3), 200-206.

Dorheim, S. K., Bondevik, G. T., Eberhard-Gran, M., & Bjorvatn, B. (2009). Subjective and objective sleep among depressed and non-depressed postnatal women. *Acta Psychiatrica Scandinavia, 119,* 128-136.

Duijts, L., Jaddoe, V. V. W., Hofman, A., & Moll, H. A. (2010). Prolonged and exclusive breastfeeding reduces the risk of infectious diseases in infancy. *Pediatrics, 126,* e18-e25. doi:10.1542/peds.2008-325

Dumitriu, D., Emeruwa, U. N., Hanft, E., Liao, G. V., Ludwig, E., & Walzer, L. (2020). Outcomes of neonates born to mothers with Severe Acute Respiratory Syndrome Coronavirus 2 infection at a large medical center in New York City. *JAMA Pediatrics.* doi:10.1001/jamapediatrics.2020.4298

Dunn, N. (2009). Oral contraceptives and venous thromboembolism. *British Medical Journal, 339*(7720), 521-522.

Dvorak, B. (2010). Milk epidermal growth factor and gut protection. *Journal of Pediatrics, 156*, S1-S5. doi:10.1016/j.peds.2009.11.018

Evans, S. S., Repasky, E. A., & Fisher, D. T. (2015). Fever and the thermal regulation of immunity: The immune system feels the heat. *Nature Reviews in Immunology, 15*(6), 335-349. doi:0.1038/nri3843

Fava, C., & Montagnana, M. (2018). Atherosclerosis in an inflammation disease which lacks a common anti-inflammatory therapy: How human genetics can help to this issue: A narrative review. *Frontiers in Immunology, 9.* doi:https://doi.org/10.3389/fphar.2018.00055

Gaillard, T., Briolant, S., Madamet, M., & Pradines, B. (2017). The end of a dogma: The safety of doxycycline use in young children for malaria treatment. *Malaria Journal, 16*, 148. doi:10.1186/s12936-017-1797-9

Gould, S. J. (1996). *The mismeasure of man:* W.W. Norton.

Gunderson, E. P., Hurston, S. R., Lo, J. C., Crites, Y., Walton, D., & Dewey, K. G. (2015). Lactation and progression to type 2 diabetes mellitus after gestational diabetes mellitus. *Annals of Internal Medicine, 162*, 889-898. doi:10.7326/M15-08

Gustafsson, L., Hallgren, O., Mossberg, A.-K., Pettersson, J., Fischer, W., Aronsson, A., & Svanberg, C. (2005). HAMLET kills tumor cells by apoptosis: Structure, cellular mechanisms, and therapy. *Journal of Nutrition, 135*, 1299-1303.

Hahn-Holbrook, J., Saxbe, D. E., Bixby, C., Steele, C., & Glynn, L. M. (2019). Human milk as "chrononutrition": Implications for child health and development. *Pediatric Research, 85*, 936-942. doi:10.1038/s41390-019-0368-x

Hale, T. W., Kendall-Tackett, K. A., & Cong, Z. (2018). Domperidone versus metoclopramide: Self-reported side effects in a large sample of breastfeeding mothers who used these medications to increase milk production. *Clinical Lactation, 9*(1), 10-17.

Hansen, R., Gibson, S., de Paiva Alves, E., Goddard, M., MacLaren, A., & Karcher, A. M. (2018). Adaptive response of neonatal sepsis-derived Group B Streptococcus to bilirubin. *Scientific Reports, 8*, 6470. doi:10.1038/s41598-018-24811-3

Health Canada, Canadian Paediatric Society, Dietitians of Canada, & Breastfeeding Committee for Canada. (2014). Nutrition for healthy term infants: Recommendations from 6 to 24 months. Retrieved from https://www.canada.ca/en/health-canada/services/canada-food-guide/resources/infant-feeding/nutrition-healthy-term-infants-recommendations-birth-six-months/6-24-months.html

Hegarty, S. (2012). The myth of the eight-hour sleep. *BBC News.* Retrieved from https://www.bbc.com/news/magazine-16964783

Hewlett, B. S., & Winn, S. (2014). Allomaternal nursing in humans. *Current Anthropology, 55*(2), 200-229.

Hoseth, E., Joergensen, A., Ebbesen, F., & Moeller, M. (2000). Blood glucose levels in a population of healthy, breast fed, term infants of appropriate sixe for gestational age. *Archives of Disease of Childhood Fetal and Neonatal Edition, 83*, F117-F119.

International Labour Organization. (2012). Allow moms to breastfeed at work. Retrieved from https://www.ilo.org/global/about-the-ilo/newsroom/news/WCMS_186325/lang--en/index.htm

Jasani, B., Simmer, K., Patole, S. K., & Rao, S. C. (2017). Long-chain polyunsaturated fatty acid supplementation in infants born at term. *Cochrane Database of Systematic Reviews*. Retrieved from https://doi.org/10.1002/14651858.CD000376.pub4

Jernstrom, H., Lubinski, J., Lynch, P., Ghardirian, L. P., Neuhausen, S., & Isaacs, C. (2004). Breastfeeding and the risk of breast cancer in BRCA1 and BRCA2 mutation carriers. *Journal of the National Cancer Institute, 96*(14), 1094-1098. doi:10.1093/jnci/djh211

Johannes, C. B., Varas-Lorenzo, C., McQuay, L. J., Midkiff, K. D., & Fife, D. (2010). Risk of serious ventricular arrhythmia and sudden cardiac death in a cohort of users of domperidone: A nested case-control study. *Pharmacoepidemiology and Drug Safety, 19*(9), 881-888. doi:10.1002/pds.2016

Johnson, C. L., & Versalovic, J. (2012). The human microbiome and its potential importance to pediatrics. *Pediatrics, 129*, 950. doi:10.1542/peds.2011-2736

Jung, C. (2015, Oct 16). Overselling breastfeeding. *New York Times*. Retrieved from https://www.nytimes.com/2015/10/18/opinion/sunday/overselling-breast-feeding.html

Kapp, N., & Curtis, K. M. (2010). Combined oral contraceptive use among breastfeeding women: A systematic review. *Contraception, 82*, 10-16. doi:10.1016/j.contraception.2010.02.001

Kendall-Tackett, K. A., Cong, Z., & Hale, T. W. (2011). The effect of feeding method on sleep duration, maternal well-being, and postpartum depression. *Clinical Lactation, 2*(2), 22-26.

Khazan, O. (2020). The ominous rise of toddler milk. *The Atlantic*. Retrieved from //www.theatlantic.com/health/archive/2020/02/should-you-buy-toddler-milk/606028/

Kundar, A. R., Singh, I., & Bulmer, A. C. (2015). Bilirubin, platelet activation and heart disease: A missing link to cardiovascular protection in Gilbert's syndrome? *Artherosclerosis, 239*, 73-84. doi:https://doi.org/10.1016/j.atherosclerosis.2014.12.042

Laing, I. A., & Wong, C. M. (2002). Hypernatraemia in the first few days: Is the incidence rising? *Archives of Disease of Childhood Fetal and Neonatal Edition, 87*, F158-F162.

Lee, H., Padhi, E., Hasegawa, Y., Larke, J., Parenti, M., Wang, A., . . . Slupsky, C. (2018). Compositional dynamics of the milk fat globule and its role in infant development. *Frontiers in Pediatrics, 6*. Retrieved from https://doi.org/10.3389/fped.2018.00313

Lerner, S. (2015). The real war on families: Why the U.S. needs paid leave now. *In these times*. Retrieved from https://inthesetimes.com/article/the-real-war-on-families

Li, R., Dee, D., Li, C.-M., Hoffman, H. J., & Grummer-Strawn, L. M. (2014). Breastfeeding and risk of infections at 6 years. *Pediatrics, 134*, S13. doi:10.1542/peds.2014-0646D

Lien, E. R., & Shattuck, K. (2017). Breastfeeding education and support services provided to family medicine and obstetrics-gynecology residents. *Breastfeeding Medicine, 12*(9), 548-553. doi:10.1089/bfm.2017.0014

Liese, A. D., Hirsch, T., von Mutius, E., Keil2001, U., Lupold, W., & Weiland, S., K. (2001). Inverse association of overweight and breastfeeding in 9 to 10-y-old children in Germany. *International Journal of Obesity, 25*, 1644-1650.

Lott, M., Callahan, E., Welker Duffy, E., Story, M., & Daniels, S. (2019). *Healthy beverage consumption in early childhood: Recommendations from key national health and nutrition organizations. Consensus statement.* Durham, NC.

Lugli, L., Bedetti, L., Lucaccioni, L., Gennari, W., Leone, C., Ancora, G., & Berardi, A. (2020). An uninfected preterm newborn inadvertently fed SARS-CoV-2-positive breast milk. *Pediatrics, 147*(4), e2020004960. doi:10.1542/peds.2020-004960

Mandel, D., Lubetzky, R., Dollberg, S., Barak, S., & Mimouni, F. B. (2005). Fat and energy contents of expressed human breast milk in prolonged lactation. *Pediatrics, 116*, e432. doi:10.1542/peds.2005-031

Marin-Gabriel, M. A., Cuadrado, I., Fernandez, B. A., Carrasco, E. G., Diaz, C. A., & Martin, I. L. (2020). Multicentre Spanish study found no incidences of viral transmission in infants borth to mothers with COVID-19. *Acta Paediatrica, 109*, 2302-2308. doi: 10.1111/apa.1547

McKechnie, A. C., & Eglash, A. (2010). Nipple shields: A review of the literature. *Breastfeeding Medicine, 5*(6), 309-314. doi:10.1089/bfm.2010.0003

McKenna, J. J. (2020). *Safe infant sleep: Expert answers to your cosleeping questions.* Washington, DC: Platypus Media.

McKinney, C. M., Glass, R. P., Coffey, P., Rue, T., Vaughn, M. G., & Cunningham, M. (2016). Feeding neonates by cup: A systematic review of the literature. *Maternal & Child Health Journal, 20*(8), 1620-1633. doi:10.1007/s10995-016-1961-9

MD BriefCase. (2021). Infant nutrition: Balancing the building blocks of brain development and immune support. Retrieved from https://www.mdbriefcase.com/course/infant-nutrition-balancing-the-building-blocks-of-brain-development-and-immune-support/

Mitoulas, L. R., Kent, J. C., Cox, D. B., Owens, R. A., Sherriff, J. L., & Hartmann, P. E. (2002). Variation in fat, lactose and protein in human milk over 24h and throughout the first year of lactation. *British Journal of Nutrition, 88*, 29-37. doi:10.1079/BJN2002579

Moises, E. C. D., Duarte, L. D. B., Cavalli, R. D. C., Lanchote, V. L., Durate, G., & de Cunha, S. P. (2005). Pharmacokinetics and transplacental distribution of fentanyl in epidural anesthesia for normal pregnant women. *European Journal of Clinical Pharmacology, 61*, 517-522. doi:10.1007/s00228-005-0967-9

Montgomery, S. M., Ehlin, A., & Sacker, A. (2006). Breast feeding and resilience against psychosocial stress. *Archives of Diseases of Childhood, 91*, 990-994.

Mosko, S., Richard, C., & McKenna, J. J. (1997a). Infant arousals during mother-infant bed sharing: Implications for infant sleep and sudden infant death syndrome research. *Pediatrics, 100*, 841-849.

Mosko, S., Richard, C., & McKenna, J. J. (1997b). Maternal sleep and arousals during bedsharing with infants. *Sleep, 20*(2), 142-150.

Munblit, D., Perkin, M. R., Palmer, D. J., Allen, K. J., & Boyle, R. (2020). Assessment of evidence about common infant symptoms and cow's milk allergy. *JAMA Pediatrics, 174*(6), 599-608. doi:10.1001/jamapediatrics.2020.0153

Narvey, M., & Canadian Paediatric Society Fetus and Newborn Committee. (2021). Breastfeeding and COVID-19. Retrieved from https://cps.ca/en/documents/position/breastfeeding-when-mothers-have-suspected-or-proven-covid-19

Newman, J. (2021). Protocol to increase breastmilk intake. Retrieved from https://ibconline.ca/information-sheets/protocol-to-increase-breastmilk-intake/

Nyqvist, K. H., Anderson, G. C., Bergman, N. J., Cattaneo, A., Charpak, N., & Davanzo, R. (2010). Towards universal Kangaroo Mother Care: Recommendations and report from the First European conference and Seventh International Workshop on Kangaroo Mother Care. *Acta Paediatrica, 99*, 820-826. doi:I:10.1111/j.1651-2227.2010.01787.x

Oddy, W. (2012). Infant feeding and obesity risk in the child. *Breastfeeding Review, 20*(2), 7-12.

Oddy, W. (2017). Breastfeeding, childhood asthma, and allergic disease. *Annals of Nutrition and Metabolism, 70*(Suppl 2), 26-36. doi:10.1159/000457920

Oddy, W. H., Kendall, G. E., Li, J., Jacoby, P., Robinson, M., de Klerk, N. H., . . . Stanley, F. J. (2009). The long-term effects of breastfeeding on child and adolescent mental health: A pregnancy cohort study followed for 14 years. *Journal of Pediatrics, 156*(4), 568-574.

Oropeza, L. G., Rosado, J. L., Ronquillo, D., Garcia, O. P., Caamano, M. D. C., Garcia-Ugalde, C., . . . Duarte-Vazquez, M. A. (2018). Lower protein intake supports normal growth of full-term infants fed formula: A randomized controlled trial. *Nutrients, 10*, 886. doi:10.3390/nu10070886

Osband, Y. B., Altman, R. L., Patrick, P. A., & Edwards, K. S. (2011). Breastfeeding education and support services offered to pediatric residents in the US. *Academic Pediatrics, 11*(1), 75-79. doi:10.1016/j.acap.2010.11.002

Pace, R. M., Williams, J. E., Jarvinen, K. M., Belfort, M. B., Pace, C. D. W., Lackey, K. A., & Gogle, A. (2021). Characterization of SARS-CoV-2 RNA, antibodies, and neutralizing capacity in milk produced by women with COVID-19. *mBio, 12*(1), e03192-03120. doi:10.1128/mBio.03192-20

Patro-Golab, B., Zalewski, B. M., Kouwenhoven, S. M. P., Karas, J., Koletzko, B., van Goudoever, J. B., & Szajewska, H. (2016). Protein concentration in milk formula, growth, and later risk of obesity: A systematic review. *Journal of Nutrition, 146*, 551-564. doi:10.3945/jn.115.223651

Paulaviciene, I. J., Liubsys, A., Molyte, A., Eidukaite, A., & Usonis, V. (2020). Circadian changes in the composition of human milk macronutrients depending on pregnancy duration: A cross-sectional study. *International Breastfeeding Journal, 15*(49). Retrieved from https://doi.org/10.1186/s13006-020-00291-y

Price, A. M. H., Wake, M., Ukoumunne, O. G., & Hiscock, H. (2012). Five-year follow-up of harms and benefits of behavioral infant sleep intervention: Randomized trial. *Pediatrics, 130*(4), 643-651. Retrieved from www.pediatrics.org/cgi/doi/10.1542/peds.2011-3467

Quigley, M. A., Hockley, C., Carson, C., Kelly, Y., Renfrew, M., & Sacker, A. (2012). Breastfeeding is associated with improved child cognitive development: A population-based cohort study. *Journal of Pediatrics, 160*, 25-32. https://doi.org/10.1016/j.jpeds.2011.06.035

Quigley, M. A., Kelly, Y. J., & Sacker, A. (2007). Breastfeeding and hospitalization for diarrheal and respiratory infection in the United Kingdom Millennium Cohort Study. *Pediatrics, 119*, 837-842. doi:10.1542/peds.2006-22

Quinn, E. A. (2014). Too much of a good thing: Evolutionary perspectives on infant formula fortification in the United States and Its effects on infant health. *American Journal of Human Biology, 26,* 10-17. doi:10.1002/ajhb.22476

Ram, K. T., Bobby, P., Hailpern, S. M., Lo, J. C., Schocken, M., Skurnick, J., & Santoro, N. (2008). Duration of lactation is associated with lower prevalence of the metabolic syndrome in midlife--SWAN, the study of women;s health across the nation. *American Journal of Obstetrics and Gynecology, 198*(3), e1-6.

Ransjo-Arvidson, A.-B., Mattiesen, A. S., Lilja, G., Nissen, E., Widstrom, A. M., & Uvnas-Moberg, K. (2001). Maternal analgesia during labor disturbs newborn behavior: Effects on breastfeeding, temperature, and crying. *Birth, 28*(1), 5-12.

Reiley, L. (2019). Sweet excess: How the baby-food industry hooks toddlers on sugar, salf, and fat. *Washington Post.* Retrieved from https://www.washingtonpost.com/business/2019/10/17/sweet-excess-how-baby-food-industry-hooks-toddlers-sugar-salt-fat/

Roberts, E. A., & Young, L. (2002). Maternal-infant transmission of Hepatitis C virus infection. *Hepatology, 36,* S106-S113. doi:10.1053/jhep.2002.36792

Sadeharju, K., Knip, M., Virtanen, S. M., Savilahti, E., Taurianen, S., Koskela, P., . . . The Finnish TRIGR Study. (2007). Maternal antibodies in breast milk protect the child from Enterovirus infections. *Pediatrics, 119,* 941-946. doi:10.1542/peds.2006-22

Sanchez-Infantes, D., Cereijo, R., Sebastiani, G., Perez-Cruz, M., Villarroya, F., & Ibanez, L. (2018). Nerve growth factor levels in term human infants: Relationship to prenatal growth and early postnatal feeding. *International Journal of Endocrinology.* Retrieved from https://doi.org/10.1155/2018/7562702

Sapolsky, R. M. (1996). Why stress is bad for your brain. *Science, 273,* 749-750.

Schwartz, E. B., Ray, R. M., Stuebe, A. M., Allison, M. A., Ness, R. B., Freiberg, M. S., & Cauley, J. A. (2009). Duration of lactation and risk factors for maternal cardiovascular disease. *Obstetrics & Gynecology, 113*(5), 974-982.

Sedlak, T. W., & Snyder, S. H. (2004). Bilirubin benefits: Cellular protection by a biliverdin reductase antioxidant cycle. *Pediatrics, 113,* 1176.

Segal, S. (2010). Labor epidural analgesia and maternal fever. *Anesthesia & Analgesia, 111,* 1467-1475. doi:10.1213/ANE.0b013e3181f73d4

Sim, K., Powell, E., Shaw, A. G., McClure, Z., Bangham, M., & Kroll, J. S. (2013). The neonatal gastrointestinal microbiota: The foundation of future health? *Archives of Disease of Childhood Fetal and Neonatal Edition, 98,* F362-F364. doi:10.1136/archdischild-2012-302872

Stage, E., Mathiesen, E. R., Emmersen, P. B., Greisen, G., & Damm, P. (2010). Diabetic mothers and their newborn infants--rooming in and neonatal morbidity. *Acta Paediatrica, 99,* 997-999. doi:10.1111/j.1651-2227.2010.01779.x

Stuebe, A. M., Rich-Edwards, J. W., Willett, W. C., Manson, J. E., & Michels, K. B. (2005). Duration of lactation and incidence of type 2 diabetes. *Journal of the American Medical Association, 294*(20), 2601-2610

Su, D., Pasalich, M., Lee, A., & Binns, C. W. (2013). Ovarian cancer risk is reduced by prolonged lactation: A case-control study in Southern China. *American Journal of Clinical Nutrition, 97,* 354-359. doi:0.3945/ajcn.112.044719

Thompson, J. M. D., Tanabe, K. O., Moon, R. Y., Mitchell, E. A., McGarvey, C., Tappin, D., . . . Hauck, F. R. (2017). Duration of breastfeeding and risk of SIDS: An individual participant data meta-analysis. *Pediatrics, 140*, e20171324. doi:https://doi. org/10.1542/peds.2017-1324

Titus-Ernstoff, L., Perez, K., Cramer, D. W., Harlow, B. L., Baron, J. A., & Greenberg, E. R. (2001). Menstrual and reproductive factors in relation to ovarian cancer risk. *British Journal of Cancer, 84*(5), 714-721. doi:10.1054/ bjoc.2000.159

Tiwari, K., Khanam, I., & Savarna, N. (2018). A study on effectiveness of lactational amenorrhea as a method of contraception. *International Journal of Reproduction, Contraception, Obstetrics, and Gynecology, 7*(10), 39463950. doi:10.18203/2320-1770. ijrcog20183837

Todd, S. R., Dahlgren, F. S., Traeger, M. S., Beltran-Aguilar, E. D., Marianos, D. W., Hamilton, C., . . . Regan, J. J. (2015). No visible dental staining in children treated with doxycycline for suspected Rocky Mountain Spotted Fever. *Journal of Pediatrics, 166*(5), 1246-1250. doi:10.1016/j.peds.2015.02.015

Torvaldsen, S., Roberts, C. L., Simpson, J. M., Thompson, J. F., & Ellwood, D. A. (2006). Intrapartum epidural analgesia and breastfeeding: A prospective cohort study. *International Breastfeeding Journal, 1*(1), 24, Retrieved from https://doi. org/10.1186/1746-4358-1-24

Tran, H. T., Nguyen, P. T. K., Huynh, L. T., Le, C. H. M., Giang, H. T. N., Nguyen, P. T., & Murray, J. (2020). Appropriate care for neonates born to mothers with COVID-19 disease. *Acta Paediatrica, 109*, 1713-1716. doi: 10.1111/apa.15413

Tromp, I., Kiefte-deJong, J., Raat, H., Jaddoe, V. V. W., Franco, O., Hofman, A., . . . Moll, H. A. (2017). Breastfeeding and the risk of respiratory tract infections after infancy: The Generation R Study. *PLoS One, 12*(2), e0172763. doi:10.1371/journal.pone.0172763

Tryggvadottir, L., Tulinius, H., Eyfjord, J. E., & Sigurvinsson, T. (2001). Breastfeeding and reduced risk of breast cancer in an Icelandic Cohort Study. *American Journal of Epidemiology, 154*(1), 37-42.

Tung, r., A.-H., Goodman, M. T., Wu, A. H., McDuffie, K., Wilkens, L. R., Kolonel, L. N., . . . Sobin, L. H. (2003). Reproductive factors and epithelial ovarian cancer risk by histologic type: A multiethnic case-control study. *American Journal of Epidemiology, 158*(7), 629-638. doi:10.1093/aje/kwg17

Ulitzsch, D., Nyman, M. K. G., & Carlson, R. A. (2004). Breast abscess in lactating women: US-guided treatment. *Radiology, 232*(2), 904-909. doi:10.1148/radiol.23230305

UNICEF. (1989). Convention on the rights of the child. Retrieved from https://www.unicef. org/child-rights-convention#learn

UNICEF, Global Nutrition Cluster, & IFE Core Group. (2022). Joint statement: Protecting maternal and child nutrition in the Ukraine conflict and refugee crisis. Retrieved from https://mail.google.com/mail/u/0?ui=2&ik=454b16524a&attid=0.1&permm sgid=msg-f:1726829910117233671&th=17f6eea7740eb407&view=att&disp=inline

van Kempen, A. A. M. W., Eskes, P. F., Nuytemans, D. H. G. M., van der Lee, J. H., Dijksman, L. M., & van Veenendallt, N. R. (2020). *New England Journal of Medicine, 382*(6), 534-544. doi:10.1056/NEJMoa190559

van Noord, C., Dieleman, J. P., van Herpen, G., Verhamme, K., & Sturkenboom, M. C. J. M. (2010). Domperidone and ventricular arrhythmia or sudden cardiac death:

A population-based case-control study in the Netherlands. *Drug Safety, 33*(11), 1003-1014. doi:10.2165/11536840-000000000-00000

Vennemann, M. M., Bajanowski, T., Brinkmann, B., Jorch, G., Yucesan, K., Sauerland, C.,... the GeSID Study Group. (2009). Does breastfeeding reduce the risk of sudden infant death syndrome. *Pediatrics, 123*, e406-e410.

Victora, C. G., Bahl, R., Barros, A. J. D., Franca, G. V. A., Horton, S., & Krasevec, J. (2016). Breastfeeding in the 21st century: Epidemiology, mechanisms, and lifelong effect. *Lancet, 387*, 475-490. doi:10.1016/S0140-6736(15)01024-7

Widstrom, A. M., Lilja, G., Aaltomaa-Michalias, P., Dahllof, A., Lintula, M., & Nissen, E. (2011). Newborn behaviour to locate the breast when skin-to-skin: A possible method for enabling early self-regulation. *Acta Paediatrica, 100*(1), 79-85. doi:10.1111/j.1651-2227.2010.01983.x

Wiklund, I., Norman, M., Uvnas-Moberg, K., Ransjo-Arvidson, A.-B., & Andolf, E. (2009). Epidural analgesia: Breastfeeding success and related factors. *Midwifery, 25*, E31-E38. doi:10.1016/j.midw.2007.07.005

World Health Organization. (2003). Kangaroo mother care: A practical guide. Retrieved from https://apps.who.int/iris/bitstream/handle/10665/42587/9241590351. pdf?sequence=1&isAllowed=y

World Health Organization. (2010). WHO guidelines on HIV and infant feeding. Retrieved from https://apps.who.int › FWC_MCA_12.1_eng.pdf

World Health Organization. (2020). Breastfeeding and COVID-19. Retrieved from https://www.who.int/news-room/commentaries/detail/breastfeeding-and-covid-19

World Health Organization. (2021). Infant and young child feeding. Retrieved from https://www.who.int/news-room/fact-sheets/detail/infant-and-young-child-feeding

Yan, J., Liu, L., Zhu, Y., Huang, G., & Wang, P. P. (2014). The association between breastfeeding and childhood obesity: A meta-analysis. *BMC Public Health, 14*, 1267. doi:https://doi.org/10.1186/1471-2458-14-1267

Made in United States
Troutdale, OR
08/17/2023

12142260R00166